TABLE OF CONTENTS

Table of Contents………………………………... Page i
Dedication and Acknowledgements……… Page ii
Important Notice……………………………… Page iv
Chapter 1: This is My Story………………… Page 1
Chapter 2: You Are Not Alone…………… Page 5
Chapter 3: The Balancing Act……………... Page 10
Chapter 4: Diets, What's Out There?…….. Page 17
Chapter 5: Who Are You? ………………….. Page 22
Chapter 6: Calories, Calories, Calories … Page 29
Chapter 7: What About Carbs? ………….. Page 33
Chapter 8: Darned Processed Foods…… Page 43
Chapter 9: Imagine - Boat Life…………… Page 46
Chapter 10: Our Galley…………………….. Page 52
Chapter 11: Recipes………………………….. Page 57
Chapter 12: Interviews ……………………… Page 140
Chapter 13: Can I Help You? ……………. Page 187
Chapter 14: Closing Thoughts …………… Page 189
Recipes at Your Fingertips………………….. Page 192

DEDICATION AND ACKNOWLEDGEMENTS

I would first like to dedicate *Time to Stop the Battle (Eating with Freedom)* to my Mom, Frances Buono. Her words throughout the years have inspired me for the premise of this book. So often my Mom would say, "Have a little bit -- a little bit is not going to hurt you." I heard that as a little child when I didn't want to eat what was put in front of me. It taught me to stretch my taste buds and try new foods. And of course, she dealt with me through ALL my diets in my later years. I was faithful to my diet plans...until I wasn't. My mother often heard me say, "I can't eat that, Mom. It's not on my diet." And she would reply, "Every once in a while, it won't hurt you to have some." And... she would always follow with these words of encouragement, "But that's okay, Michele, you have to do what you feel you have to do."

You are going to see my Mom throughout the pages of *Time to Stop the Battle (Eating with Freedom)*. Thanks, Mom. It would take another book just to share your strength, determination and the precious love that you taught and showered on us through the years.

Love you to the moon and back! Michelly

I would next like to thank my awesome husband, Captain Steve Legge. Thank you for your support, co-writing, and editing patience. My heart belongs to you always and forever. I am ever grateful for your suggestion to put this journey on paper so that others would have the opportunity to change their lives and health as it has helped you.

I would like to give a shout of thanks to those who shared their strengths and intimate weaknesses, their successes and failures.

Your input was so important to the concept of what this book is about, people helping people through their personal experiences.

To Susan, Lupe, Karen S., Kindra, Cindy and Al, Olga, Darlene, Kathy and Peter, Patty, Rosalie, Tona, Kristie, Sophia, N.Y. Karen, Tina Peterson and Pastor Anthony Storino. Thank you for your helpful contributions to my efforts.

To my sisters Darlene and Patty who consistently supported me from page 1 and before that.

To Sue Fraga Leotteau, Doris Sanders and Cindy Panigal for the selfless time spent editing, correcting and your many suggestions that improved and made what I had written a book that flows with ease.

I appreciate all of you so much.
From my heart,
Thank you again

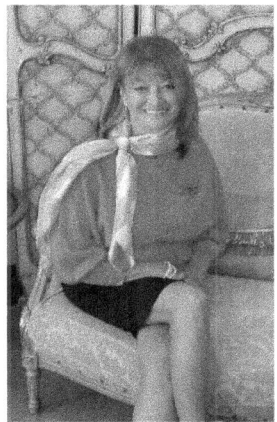

Michele

IMPORTANT NOTICE:

This book was created to share with others our experiences and years of trial and error, along with our failures and successes. Michele has no official culinary training and no formal training in the field of nutrition as well as no training as a dietitian. This book is to be used only as a reference, not as a medical manual of any kind. The information contained in this book is provided to show what we have discovered in order to take care of our personal dietary needs and meet our personal goals, and to help others in their searches for what will work for them. I have gathered the information contained in this book from a combination of sources: available diet plans, listening to other people's experience with their individual "battle of the foods," the internet, and our personal experiences.

References to various brand name products of any kind, to diet plans, establishments, companies and/or organizations are for informational purposes only. Their mention in this book does not constitute an endorsement of any kind or sponsorship of any kind.

It is recommended that, before beginning any diet or dietary change, you consult with your physician. I will not be liable for issues arising as the result of poor personal choices in diet alterations.

> *The best and most beautiful things in this world cannot be seen or even heard but must be felt with the heart.*
>
> *Helen Keller*

Chapter One - *This is My Story*

Hi, my name is Michele Legge. This is **my** crazy battle of the foods story. Everybody has one… A story, I mean.

Up until I was in my early 20's, I ate food because it was necessary to eat. I was never really hungry. I just ate because it was the time of day to eat. And, of course, I was skinny. As a teenager, one of my nicknames was Twig or Twiggy. My mom tried to help by preparing a milkshake for me every night. Oh, my goodness, they were sooo good. But after a week, I began to dread this delicious 16 oz. cup of yummy ice cream, bananas, whipped cream, and other goodies that my Mom would put into a blender in order to create a shake for me to gain weight. Finally, I just couldn't take another sip. So that was that.

But something happened during my middle 20's. I somehow acquired an appetite, an appetite that couldn't be satisfied. I don't know where it came from or why, but there it was. I would wake up in the middle of the night and down half of a chocolate cake. And I would do it often. I was hungry all of the time. And still, I was skinny.

At around 32, something new started to happen. The number on the scale suddenly started moving upwards. I was finally getting some meat on my Twiggy bones but was continually hungry. Life is so funny and crazy sometimes. Suddenly, I was now on the other side. Now I was trying to keep the scale number in the same place. This was the beginning... and so my diets began.

Time to Stop the Battle (Eating with Freedom) is about this phase in my life of dieting and what I learned and took away from each diet plan I tried. And let me tell you…there were a lot of them to take from. Frequently throughout the pages of this book you will see words repeated over and over. Words such as:

>Diet
>Choices
>Moderation
>Modification
>And the very important...."yum"

You will also see phrases like "moderate and modify" or "what works for you" and "what are the foods you enjoy," plus a few more that target your personal needs and taste buds.

But this is not just a story about me, it is a story about my husband as well. When we met in 1984, he weighed about 172 pounds and wore size 32 jeans. Well, over the years he steadily gained weight until at 234 pounds and tight size 42 jeans; after two visits to the emergency room within a week with Atrial Fibrillation (A-fib: rapid and irregular beating of the atria); 1 minor heart attack followed by 3 stents placed in his arteries and out of control diabetes (with yet another strong request from his doctor to lose some weight), my husband asked me to support him in his efforts to drop those numbers with the intention of trying to improve his health. Throughout this book I will share with you the great education that my own dieting experiences provided for that effort. Because of the things I learned while in my dieting season, I was able to adapt changes into my husband's eating habits. All of these "personal adaptations" have produced what I believe to be remarkable results. My husband will tell you a little about his experience later in the book. But (spoiler alert), Steve loves the results of his new eating habits. Today at 180 pounds he asked me to write about it and so ***Time to Stop the Battle (Eating with Freedom)*** was birthed.

When he asked me to help him with his goal to lose the excess weight, I reflected back on all of the diets I that had tried in the past that worked for me. There were many I liked and appreciated. What was it about each one that I liked and appreciated? I don't think it needs to be said, but the nutritional value of each meal had to be acceptable to me. That is something which needs to be considered in every search for a diet. However, equally as important, (and I believe even more important) were the following two major considerations:

- I had to enjoy what I was eating and…
- I definitely did not want to be hungry

That's what worked for me. So, the question I started with was, "What foods does my husband like to eat?" Everybody should start with a similar question. The answer will give you some direction. What are the foods that you enjoy? My starting place was fast food. Steve is a burger and fries' type of guy and I knew that this was where I needed to begin. That is what this book is about. It is about **you** and what **you** like to eat.

You need to find your own way and my hope is that our experience and tips will help you find your freedom with eating. And so, our story continues…

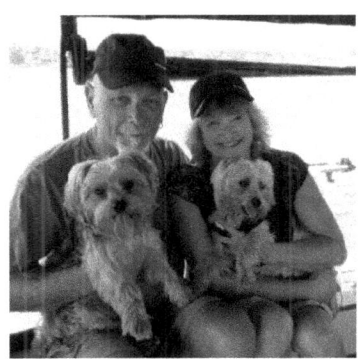

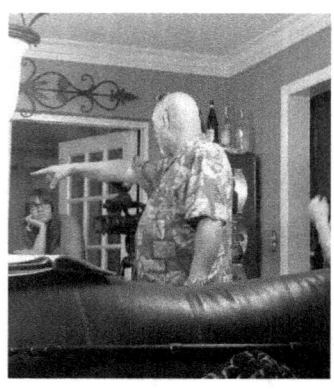 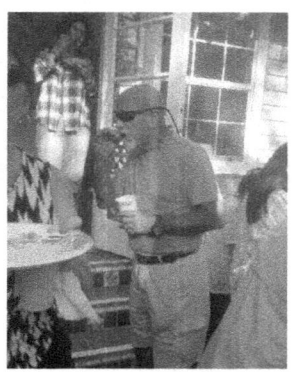

Steve Before at 234 lbs.   Steve After at 180 lbs.

Every day is a new chance…a new beginning!

Chapter 2 -- *You Are Not Alone!*

It is extremely important for you to know that you are not alone. You're not the only one with a food battle. I believe the greater majority of people fight the food battle every day just as you and I do. Truth be told, there are very few people that have a tiny, perfect body because of their genetics.

I recently chatted with a high school bestie of mine. We have been friends for over 40 years. Karen was always slim. My intention was to ask her if she would participate in an interview that I was doing with others. So I asked her what her plan of attack had been with food. She told me she really had no plan to speak of for me to ask questions about. She said, "At 101 pounds, it's not all that great not having some meat on your bones." She went on to say that when she eats a lot, she may gain 10 pounds and then she just loses them. It just goes. And on those days where she may not be feeling great and a loss of appetite occurs, again, she loses. Although I am sure many of you would like to have her issues, Karen made it very clear, an issue is an issue and that she also engages in the great battle of foods...just in a different direction. Thanks for sharing with us, Karen.

Emotional eating is something that needs to be addressed. Common causes of emotional eating include "stuffing emotions." Eating can be a way to temporarily silence or "stuff down" uncomfortable emotions such as anger, fear, sadness, anxiety, loneliness, resentment, and shame. There is also nervous eating and eating as the result of depression.

Were you able to relate to any of these common causes as you read through them? Only you can answer that question. Only you know their severity. And only you can decide whether you need outside help or not. But I can tell you this... you are not alone. Everyone is emotionally connected with food. If there is a celebration, there is food. If there is drama or tragedy, there is always someone in place saying, "You need to eat, you need to keep up your strength." Everyone has experienced an emotional connection with food on some level. You are not alone!

I was discussing *Time to Stop the Battle (Eating with Freedom)* with Kindra, a liveaboard boater friend of mine. She mentioned that she would like to lose some weight. As our conversation continued, she also said that she never eats everything that is on her plate. She shared that it was because of an abusive issue that she dealt with as a child. As a child she was forced to finish everything that was set before her. At times, the forcing would get quite physical. Emotional scars were formed at the dinner table. Today, as an adult, it's just an automatic thing for her to leave a bite of food on her plate.

As a child, my mother's expectation was that we would finish what was on our plate as well. That was also my expectation with my children. But unlike Kindra, it was not an emotionally harsh experience. And I believe, for most, it is a healthy thing to leave a bit of food behind. It is a sign of control. A control that is helpful with food addictions.

We all have a story. Be okay with being a human being. You are not alone. If you recognize that you are an emotional eater, try to establish new habits. I do this every day to this very day. I don't put anything in my galley cabinets (boat kitchen) or pantry that I know that I tend to lack control over the amount that I eat, like cereal!

"We" are not alone would be more accurate for the title of this chapter. The following are some of my practices that I would like you to consider.

- Realize which foods give you a chewing satisfaction.

- Don't let hunger overwhelm you. Plan appropriate snacks ahead of time and eat them before hunger attacks.
- Plan that mid-day fill in. The great majority of fruits and veggies are low in calories. Munch away… (Fruit juices do not apply here due to the high sugar content which is equal to far too many added calories.)
- You may be an evening snacker, as are we. Morning, mid-morning, mid-afternoon, evening and even middle-of-the-night hunger pangs happen. Feeling guilty or feeling like a failure because you want something to eat does not take away that pang. Again, plan something to eat and be ready if this occurs.

IT IS WHAT YOU EAT THROUGHOUT THE DAY – NOT WHEN YOU EAT IT.

We make choices every minute of every day. When to get up, what to wear, what the agenda will be for the day *and* what we eat! Can you put your eating habits into a "choice" category? Realizing the personal choices we make through the day empowers us to make changes.

We live in a fast-paced world. This fast pace has invaded our nutritional refueling time. I can hear the echo of my mother's voice, "Slow down, Michele." I must confess that this is a difficult one for me. To this day, I inhale my food. I believe that I am not alone in this bad habit either. Working, raising children, or taking care of a home after work for both men and women sometimes makes it difficult at times to take things down to a slower pace.

Eating is, more often than not, treated as an inconvenience. Stopping to eat may hold us up from what we think are more important things to do or accomplish. We tend to focus on the busy and not nourishment. Is this you? It is almost silly to think how most people are so obsessed with food and yet we don't stop to enjoy, taste, and reap the benefits of our meals.

Studies have shown the benefits of eating slower:

- A probable decrease in food consumption therefore preventing overeating.
- Chewing food more completely leads to better appetite regulation and improved satiety.
- Better digestion.
- Better hydration.
- Easier weight loss or maintenance.
- Greater satisfaction with the meal.

Whereas, eating quickly leads to:
- Poor digestion.
- Increased weight gain.
- Lower meal satisfaction.

Consciously chewing food longer will slow down the amount of food you consume, improving the nutritional value and aiding in weight loss. So try taking smaller bites. Take the time to chew your food and swallow completely before taking another bite. It is also suggested to wait until your swallow is completed before drinking fluids.

This would logically bring me to the benefits of drinking water.

- It boosts your metabolism.
- Cleanses your body of waste.
- Acts as an appetite suppressant.
- Helps your body stop retaining water, aiding you in dropping those extra pounds of water weight.
- Flushes toxins from the body.
- Improves skin complexion.
- Increases energy and relieves fatigue.

Experts recommend that we drink at least eight 8-ounce glasses per day which is 2 liters or a half gallon. I have found that our "Sodastream" has been very helpful in increasing the amount of water that we drink daily. We enjoy the sparkling water that it provides. As a result, we drink more water.

So, right again Mom! I do enjoy my meals more when I take the time to taste what is on my plate. When I take the time to enjoy the taste of my meal, my body is given a chance to digest properly and I don't eat as much.

It is really a simple thing to try. Eat slower and drink the recommended amount of water. Personally, I have the water thing down pat, but I have to thoughtfully and intentionally work on eating slower. I am better at it than I used to be, and I can feel the difference when I heed my mom's advice.

Everyone makes daily choices. It's just that for some people it's such an immense struggle to make the right choice, which makes it begin to feel like a losing battle. They just give up and eat whatever they want. Everyone must find a way that works for them…EVERYONE…Make a decision to search and find your way today.

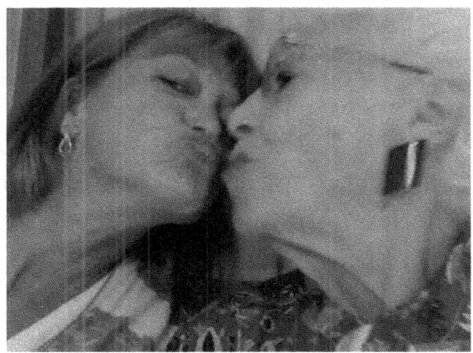

Mom & Me

Chapter 3 -- *The Balancing Act*

As I did my research and thought about what I wanted to share with you, honestly, I felt overwhelmed. **"Eating better... where do I start?"** There are some websites that promote eating protein and fats. Other sites are saying eat lots of veggies, and don't forget fruit. Wait a minute! Fruit is full of sugar! Is that the GOOD sugar or the BAD sugar? Oh yes, eat the fruit, it's good for you. Don't drink the fruit. There is more sugar in fruit juices. Some plans suggest just eating berries for your fruit intake. Processed foods are bad for you...No, maybe not...I read a site that said that overly refined processed foods are the ones that are bad. There are those who think that calorie-counting is a thing of the past and others say that it's alive and well. Dropping that extra weight can be so overwhelming and such a task, especially when sorting through all the online opinions of what is good for weight loss and what isn't.

I am not qualified to tell you what to eat or not to eat, but I am qualified to share our personal journey. I have found that our personal journey is more of a combination of the different things that I have researched. I believe that balance is an important aspect in every area of our lives. Keep balance in mind as you investigate dietetic studies.

THE DEFINITION OF A BALANCED DIET

A balanced diet is a diet that contains the proportions of carbohydrates, fats, proteins, minerals and water that are all necessary to maintain good health.

Courage is fear that has said its' prayers and decided to go forward anyway.
Joyce Meyer

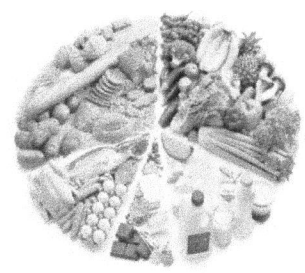

HEALTHY EATING DEFINED

Eating a variety of foods that give you the nutrients that your body requires to maintain your health, feel good, and have energy: that's healthy eating.

You are well on your way to finding a way that works for you. You are searching. That is how you came across our journey. Most everyone starts with a search; you are ready to make those modifications needed for your health. I believe you are aware that whatever path you find, your chosen "goal getter" will only work, if you work it! That is why I stress again and again, "Who are you? Which path do you feel you can be faithful to?" In the end, it may not be the most popular diet of the day!

When you come across a plan that sounds like it is the one for you, don't just try it…DO IT! Be excited and get started. And if you find out that it's not what you thought it would be or that there were too many restrictions for you to be comfortable with, don't be discouraged. You are well ahead of when you first started. Use that plan as a stepping stone. Ask yourself what it was that attracted you to that particular plan. Use both the positive and negative information you find to be of help in continuing your search.

You have and will continue to see "moderate and modify" very often. It simply means balance. Using my Italian upbringing with pasta dishes for example... many of our meals through the week were pasta based. Every Sunday, my mom would start her day by putting a pot of sauce on the stove to slow cook while we were at church. Mmmm, we would walk in the door from church and the aroma filtered right through our noses to our taste buds. I could actually taste it. I remember hovering around the kitchen until mom completed the rest of the meal. I believe impatient was the word. Our plates would have pasta covered in sauce, with a meatball, maybe a piece of sausage and some days, bigoli. We would have a loaf of sliced Italian bread on the table. And that was for scooping up all the extra sauce on our plate. There was an abundance of spaghetti before us and we were always encouraged to have that second plate. And of course, we did. This meal was off-balance. It needed to be modified and moderated. It was tilted with an overload of carbs. But this doesn't mean you can't eat it. The meal just needed balance.

In the Recipe Chapter of this book, you will see my pasta dishes, where I modified and moderated. I think if you try each of these, you'll find them really yummy. To give you a sneak preview of the recipes, one of the main problems with pasta is just this, *it's the main dish*, as I just mentioned.

I have found this to be one of the easiest dishes to modify. And that's the secret to pasta in your diet. It's just not a good idea for it to be the only food on your plate. But you don't have to do without it either, or leave the table dissatisfied and hungry.

In the world of calorie conscious folks that we are, I really need to address caloric balance. I think the following is a great example of poor caloric balance. Hypothetically, you have figured out the total amount of calories for your personal goals to be 1400 calories per day. Let's say you have decided that eating every 2 hours keeps the hunger away. If your favorite

> *The struggle in your today is developing your strength you need for tomorrow.*

donut is 200 calories each, 7 of them throughout the day would keep you at your caloric goal. But there's a problem with this logic, there is no balance. The only thing achieved would be a probable upset stomach, and sadly enough, unwanted weight gain.

What about eating out? Talk to your servers. Tell them your needs. If you don't see something suitable on the menu, ask them to modify one of their dishes for you. It is always possible. I believe you will find that in most cases they will be more than willing to help you. Part of their job is to make sure you are a happy, satisfied and hopefully a returning customer.

I have spent time on websites like *MyFittnessPal,* which provides a lot of helpful information. Another is *Lose It* (A calorie counting app.), and another is *FatSecret*. I found FatSecret to be a very easy tracker. You will find calorie trackers and goal setting on all these sites as well. You will also find out that you are eating more calories than you think you are eating. This will help you determine that balance you are looking for.

My mother says, "Too much of anything is not good for you." But being hungry is not an option, either!

These sites will also help you determine your personal choices of "fill me up" foods. Fill me up foods are a very personal part of weight loss programs. They vary according to different diet plans. For example, I don't eat many nuts. I enjoy them and eat them in moderation, but they are not a "go to" snack for me. My friend Cindy snacks on them all the time. They are a recommended snack in her diet.

I would like to address exercise and I will be brief. Balance, preference and personal needs apply with exercise as well. I am a walker. That is what I like to do. Prior to Steve's weight loss, he wasn't willing to walk. He would say that he didn't like to walk. He would always say, much to my disappointment, "Let's take the car." We would go to the grocery store and he would circle the parking lot for as long as it would take to get a front row parking space. He would walk slowly and needed to "literally" stop for a minute every couple of hundred feet or so because he claimed that he had a cramp in his leg. The truth was that he was getting chest pains. He had to stop until they subsided enough for him to continue his slow walk. Today, I almost have to look through binoculars to find the front door of the grocery store. He teases me telling me that I am the slow walker. He's got a natural get up and go today. Now, I really do have to quicken my steps when I am walking with him.

We are not people who practice a daily exercise regimen. However, we do like to walk these days and walking is very healthy for you. I just want to point out the differences. There are many who believe that exercise should accompany any weight loss plan. It is almost one word to them - "dietandexercise". Steve is off his heart, blood pressure, and cholesterol medication today. Although he was not grossly obese, it would not have been a wise choice for him, with the heart problems, to exercise along with the changes in his diet. Exercise IS very important, I'm sure all would agree, but Steve needed to drop the weight first. Everybody is different, with different sets of circumstances...

"What works for you?"

Is exercise an option for you? What type of exercise do you think you can be faithful to? Do you have any limitations, like my husband had? What do you like to eat? Find a plan that has your choices included in it and simply modify and moderate when necessary. Count those calories and determine whatever else your health needs are.

What you focus on, you become!

Put Google to work for you to fit your personal needs. Eat with freedom. We have left the "battle of food" behind us. If we want to eat it, we eat it with modification and moderation.

Go as long as you can and then take another step!

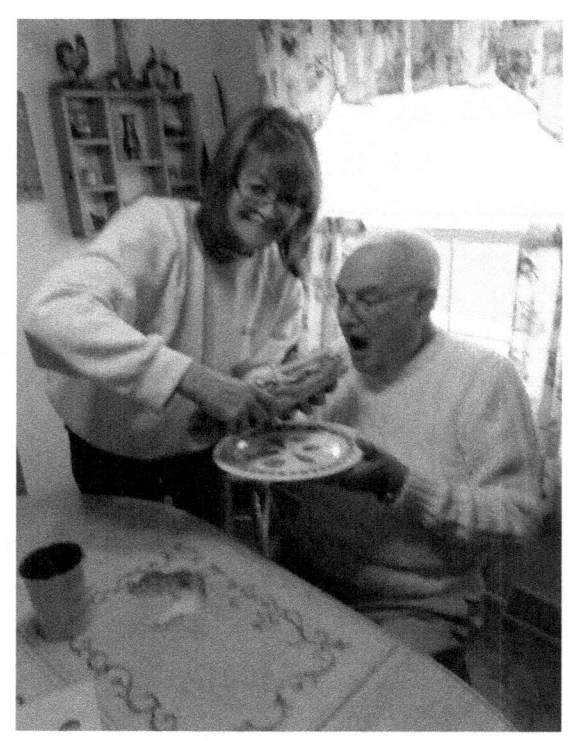

Hoagies Must Have Been the Freedom Choice of This Day!

"OPEN WIDE, POP!"

Chapter 4 -- *Diets; What's Out There*

I found that people don't like to say the word "diet". They prefer saying that it's a change of eating habits or a different way of eating. Some refer to a diet as a "life change," and it should be. Folks, the word "diet" is not a bad word. Everybody is on a diet. It's what you choose to eat. Webster's medical definition of a diet is:

1. Food and drink regularly provided or consumed.
2. Habitual nourishment.
3. The kind and amount of food prescribed for a person or animal for a special reason.
4. A regimen of eating and drinking sparingly to reduce one's weight.

That last one is what most people think of and it's the one that nobody wants to deal with, because it has the word "sparingly" in it, which equates to hunger. Let's look at numbers 1 and 2. It is simply what you eat. Our personal diet is one of choice, modification, and moderation. You choose what you want to eat and know that some foods just need to be consumed in moderation and other foods allow you to have seconds. ***Time to Stop the Battle (Eating with Freedom)*** means finding a way to eat what you enjoy without being hungry.

There are so many diets out there. Some prepare the food for you. You order it and it comes in the mail and all you have to do is eat what they send you. I have never done that, but I have, to date, only heard good things about most of them. (I have interviewed a few individuals who will help you decide if this is a good plan for you.)

Some offer supplements and others offer snacks that you can order and have delivered to your home. Some offer a partial diet, meaning that there is a drink (shake) or food bar available for one or two of your meals, and provide suggestions for your other meals. And some are a combination of all the above.

There are diets that promote exercise with their plan, and certainly exercise is a very healthy activity. There are several different herbs, natural options, and medications on the market that may assist you in curbing your appetite.

There are low carb diets, no carb diets, vegetarian diets, vegan diets and liquid protein diets. There are organic based diets and raw food diets. There is Weight Watchers, Ketogenic, Zone, Slim-Fast, Jenny Craig, South Beach, Atkins, and more. I'm pretty sure that you can add to this list. I haven't even scratched the surface. There are so many more, I could go on and on.

It seems that there are as many pre-planned diets out there as there are people searching for them. It can prove to be a crazy maze. You can find a plan that you think will work for you, talk to a friend, hear what's working for them, and find yourself right back at the start of the maze, filled with more questions than the answers you were searching for.

I have found that people tend to be very passionate in their beliefs, generally stemming from research, resulting in their chosen diets, not to mention their successful results. Because of this, I'm sure there will be those that also passionately disagree with my personal findings and research.

Most diets work if you follow the instructions, and they all have instructions. Some are healthier than others. And, of course, some are not so healthy. My question is this, because you are currently searching, which one works, or, if it be the case, worked for you? And why is it not working for you now? The answer is simple. It just wasn't a realistic life change for you. You got tired of not eating foods that you enjoy. Those foods were no longer on your list of choices according to your chosen diet plan.

One of my past chosen plans took me off fruits. And, as I believe everyone has experienced, I thought I could do without them because, after all, if I was hungry, I was given a list of foods that could take that hungry feeling away. Right? WHAT was I thinking? NO FRUIT??? SERIOUSLY??? I love fruit. I love all kinds of fruit. Telling me that I could have berries if I wanted fruit just was not ok with me. Of course, I figured that out *after* I was into the plan.

It was working, and I did enjoy my food plan until I passed the beautiful, juicy, colorful inviting fruit section in the produce department at my local grocery store. "Hmm," I thought to myself, "I've been at this plan for a while, I'm doing good, one orange can't hurt. It's just an orange." Then my brain reminded me that it's just fruit and fruit is good for you. It has vitamin-C among other things.

In a few weeks my refrigerator was full of yummy fruit again. Back to the drawing board, and a new search begins!

Another diet took my pasta away. Guys, I'm Italian! Need I say more? Well, actually, yes. I need to say more on that subject. I really enjoy zucchini noodles and I enjoy all types of pasta. But I really enjoy the pasta I grew up with. Folks, that is pasta made with white flour. This is where *modify and moderate when needed* comes into play.

Thinking that you can change who you are is absurd. But that doesn't mean that you can't make choice changes by trying new things and stretching yourself. In fact, people who stretch before their exercises find that they can push themselves a bit further. I think that is true with stretching your food choices as well.

My choices come from many diet plans. I've taken a little from each one. I have been on South Beach Diet, Weight Watchers, and Atkins. I have followed Suzanne Somers diet books. My favorite Suzanne Somers edition was *Eat Great, Lose Weight*. I love *Hungry Girl* by Lisa Lillien. I have tried the Daniel diet and followed a vegetarian diet. I've tried low-fat on my own and a few other fad diets.

I'm not promoting any of the diet plans I have been on, but I can tell you that they all worked for me. But I just didn't stick with any of them and none of them would have worked for my husband long-term. However, I did find our eating choices through them and I have an appreciation for each of them. There are many plans, of course, that I have not tried.

One of my fad diets was a delicious vegetable soup diet. Anytime I was hungry I could eat as much of it as I wanted. Oh, my goodness, it was so yummy, but by the third day, the yummy was dissipating at lightning speed. It was only a two-week plan. I didn't quite make it. I have tried so many plans where I couldn't eat this and couldn't eat that. I have often said I have grown accustomed to eating cardboard, foods with no flavor, foods that had a weird texture.

On another note, we enjoy French fries and occasionally indulge on those tasty spuds. I will either give it a go in my Nu-wave oven or we'll feast on those yummy, salty, greasy, ever luvin' fast food fries. "Occasionally." That's the heart of the book... ***Time to Stop the Battle (Eating with Freedom)***... Occasionally, when my husband and I dine out, we will eat those silly things that are truly not good for anybody. But most importantly, when we are invited out to someone's home for dinner, we don't go off our diet, we eat and enjoy

---

Mistakes are proof that you are trying.

what's in front of us without guilt. But I must remind you again of what *Mom says* all the time, "Every now and then it's not going to hurt you."

But, back to those French fries. Most of the time we really enjoy veggie straws. They are a great substitute for fries. I enjoy mine with ketchup. And they are great if you are in the mood for chips. I used to count out a serving. But now I know what a serving looks like and there is no need to count.

Because I know myself, I won't eat them straight out of the bag. If I do, I'll just keep eating them. But I find when I remove one serving from the bag and eat them, I'm satisfied. So, here's an FYI for the servers out there. I never hand my husband the bag of straws. I hand him a serving.

I am amazed at the simplicity of planning meals these days. I still use my kitchen scale on occasion. But just like the veggie straws, I can confidently judge amounts and calories. Counting what is important to us; calories, carbs, cholesterol and sodium, has become a brief review for most of our meals.

I used Google to find all of the numbers that I had to count. It was pretty simple. When you go into Google, just type "Nutritional Value of ___" and let Google do the rest of the work. You will get several sites with information, but for consistency and simplicity, look at the Wikipedia response.

Losers quit when they fail. Winners fail until they succeed!

Chapter 5-- *Who Are You?*

Let's talk about what is healthy. People are looking for the "healthy" diet. That is a number one priority, our health. Isn't that why you are searching for help, to change those numbers on the scale?

My hope, as I have said before, is that ***Time to Stop the Battle (Eating with Freedom)*** will get you where you need to go. There's always a healthier way, and certainly I'm all for that. My point here is: *let's get the weight down*. I am thoroughly convinced that after investigating for yourself, finding different recipes and foods you like to eat, searching out what works for you to lose your weight, will trigger a lifestyle, a diet that works for you. After all, we are all individuals. We are not all made the same and our stats may be different. Get the weight off and go from there.

Here are a few more questions that you might want to ask yourself. What is your culture or nationality? That is so important. You cannot deny yourself the foods you were raised on. What was served to you as a child? That's what you are more likely going to enjoy. You can't ignore that! Now, simply modify and moderate when needed and stay satisfied.

Other questions to ask yourself might be. What are your goals? What do you want to accomplish by changing the way you eat? Are there medical issues that you need to look at? Do they need to be addressed with these changes that you are NOW willing to make? How much would you like to lose weekly or monthly? What is your goal weight? Write these things down. It helps having the answers to these questions written out, so you can review them whenever these thoughts come across your mind. Goal setting should always be written down and placed in an area where you can look at them from time to time. Your answer may be, "But I know exactly what my goals are. I can remember, so I don't have to write them down anywhere." You are only fooling yourself if you think that your memory alone will cover your goals. What happens the first time that you decide in your mind to lower the bar just a little bit, so you can eat something that you really want, like a large pizza with everything on it? If you have your goals written, it is not as easy to "cheat" on them. Please know that you do NOT have to post this on your refrigerator door, but it is a good idea to have them somewhere that is readily accessible.

I'm sure you have heard the phrase "Keep it simple, stupid," or KISS. I prefer "Keep it simple, silly." You are not stupid. If this is too much to look at all at one time, just do one thing at a time. That is enough. The rest will follow as you start to see results. You can look at other needs after you start dropping some of those numbers. And dropping your weight will automatically start to take care of many of those issues like needed exercise, overall health, and wellness. I would like to encourage you. Once I got started, my findings and food choices quickly became an easy flow of information.

It was very important that my husband was happy with what he ate. Let's get real here. If you are not eating food that tastes good and you enjoy, how long do you really think that you will stick with it? If you **can't have this** or you **can't have that**, how long is it going to be before you have a little bite of what you do want? And you may think, well, that little bite didn't move the scale, so you have a little more. That little more didn't hurt either, so you have just a little bit more. Before you know it, you are right back where you started, square one and again, disappointed. I believe this is the number ONE reason why people yo-yo on diets and then claim they don't work. Or maybe weight was lost and maybe even your personal goals were met, but the numbers on the scale escalate once again. I believe this is the result of having too many things taken away while dieting. You don't have to do that.

You should consider choosing food *you* enjoy and making choices that are delicious for *your* taste buds. Prepare meals that *you* will look forward to eating and a way of eating that will not get old.

Try Googling some low-cal recipes of the foods that you enjoy. It is easy. YOU CAN DO THIS! Find your way to eating what you like. Just modify the recipes and moderate the amount that you will eat when necessary. I think you will find that spending time with Google will result in a new-found freedom. Just imagine this! Whatever you feel like eating; whatever you are yearning for, you can have it. We have found this to be true for us. But again, with modification and moderation.

Which brings me to *Who We Are*. As I mentioned, I needed to start my research with burgers for my husband. So, I discovered a great ground meat substitute at Trader Joe. A substitute that made me happy with the cholesterol and calorie count. I then purchased 96% lean ground meat. This was a great starting point for us. I use them both separately, but I also combine them for the purpose of reducing the cholesterol.

I would like to interject this thought. If you are helping a loved one, ask them from time to time about the modifications you have made. Ask them how it tastes and what they think might make it better. I did that throughout my husband's change in diet. It is so important that the food is

You are stronger than you think!

yummy! It can be really hard to listen to criticism after you have done all of your research. But it is so rewarding to achieve modified meals, snacks and desserts that you can look forward to.

Today, my husband is spoiled with his diet. I should say "we" are so spoiled. We are used to large amounts of food. That's who we are. And we are used to desserts after lunch and dinner. That's what we like. In addition, we are night time snackers! A few hours after dinner we enjoy our snacks! Yes, that was snacks, PLURAL! I can't count how many times I've been told you can't lose weight if you snack at night. "You need to stop eating after 6pm." Well, this may be true for most, but I guess we don't fall into the category of MOST. We keep our calories down, we eat a lot, we like our sweets and we are night time snackers. That is who WE are. Even with all of that silliness, Steve lost 54 pounds in 12 months or less. We are able to enjoy our night time snacks because we keep our calories lower for breakfast and lunch. This is our choice for our lifestyle. Our usual breakfast, lunch and dinner choices can be found in the recipe section of this book. I experimented with our sweets until I accomplished my caloric goals per serving. You will also find these in the recipe section of this book. These are the meals I actually prepare.

I am not suggesting that you duplicate our eating habits. I am aware that food in abundance, dessert consumption and night time snacking is not the normal format for weight loss. But please keep reading. We found our way through all of that and dropped the numbers on that dreaded scale anyway. I have to say, I have come across programs recommending that you eat 6 small meals per day. So I guess that eating and snacking on healthy choices throughout the day and between meals may not be so silly after all.

So, again, I want to ask… Who are you?

What foods were you raised on?
What do you like to eat?
YOU CAN DO THIS!

Are you ready to find your way? There is a plan out there that will work for you.

Time to Stop the Battle"(Eating with Freedom) is about who you are. Throughout this book I have shared who we are and what worked for us. I hope our experience encourages you to simply not do without. Don't fill your head with rules and have-to's. If what worked for us doesn't fit you or your lifestyle, search for a plan that does. Take notice of what foods you might need to eliminate, if any. Is it really feasible and acceptable to you to eliminate these foods long-term? Please remember this; if you are "denying" instead of "modifying," statistics say that you are not likely to stick with it, no matter how well intentioned.

The future depends on what you do today!

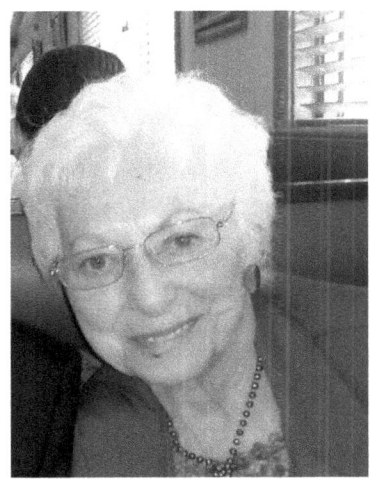
My beautiful Mom

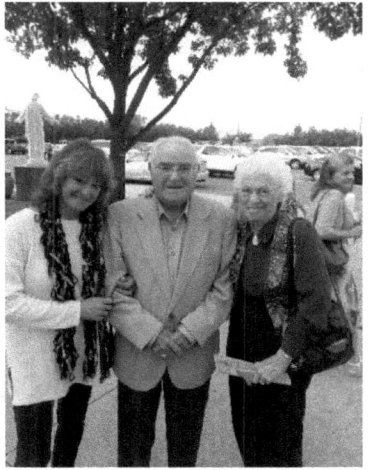
Church time with Pop and Mom

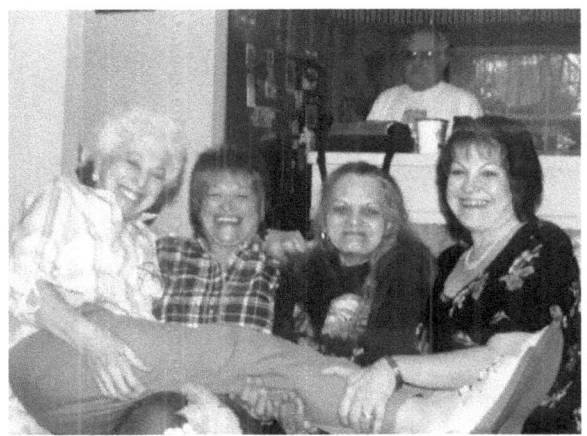
Lap time with Mom and my sisters Patty and Darlene

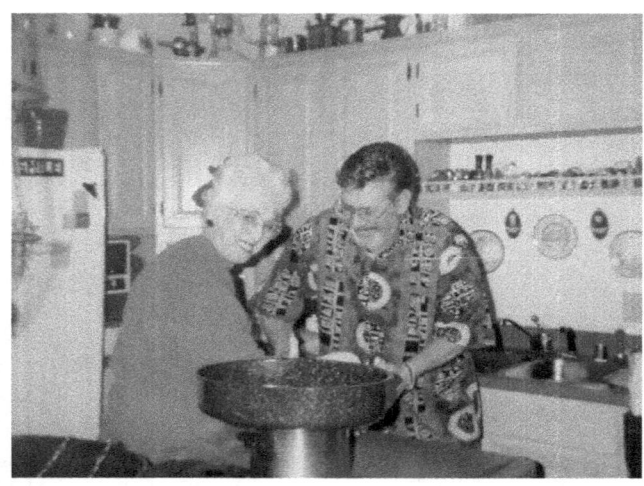

Mom and Steve having fun stuffing the turkey! Think it's still alive!

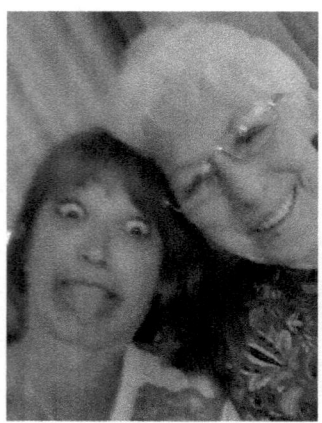

Silly willies

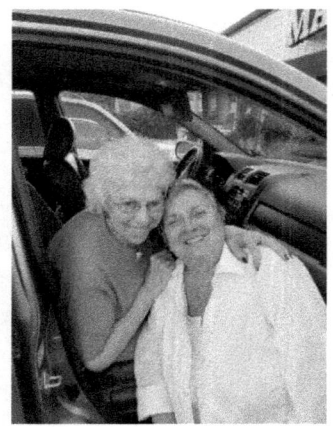

Happy faces, great visit with my cousin Theresa 2018!

Chapter 6 -- *Calories, Calories, Calories*

I started thinking about calories because, let's face it, calories play a big part in tipping the scale. Some believe that calorie counting is old school. All I can say about that is, "Welcome to my school house."

I am aware of a few plans where calories are not the main focus. But because of my husband's health issues and his food preferences, they were not a good choice for us. Actually, years back, when he first found out he was diabetic, he tried one of those diets. It did work well for a while, and, he was off his medication. While we were on vacation, he chose to eat foods that his diet plan denied him. I mean he ate anything and everything that he wanted. He chose to indulge in the wants that he hadn't had for almost a year. In the end, it threw his system so far off that he lost all of the benefits that he had gained. After our vacation, he went back to the medications and diet with a vengeance but never gained those benefits back. Truly an example of denying instead of modifying.

After calories, I went to sodium and cholesterol (sodium has been my biggest battle to keep in check). Steve had serious heart issues. I then investigated carbohydrates because of his diabetes. Today, because of technology, we have everything at our fingertips. My points of interest were all found on the internet. Time to put Google to work. The basic guidelines that I discovered for our personal plan in ***Time to Stop the Battle (Eating with Freedom)*** are throughout this book if you're not a Google user.

By now everything that I have said should tell you that I am not a dietitian or a health guru. I just read up on what's available to me on the internet concerning calories, carbs, sodium, and cholesterol. According to your health needs, you may need to add or take away from that list. Again, this is what worked for us, and the results were awesome.

Based on my research, Steve, at 5'11" and 234 pounds, needed his daily caloric intake to hover between 1800 and 2200 calories. Today, at 180 pounds or so, his daily intake hovers around 2400 calories. I am 5'6". At present, my weight fluctuates between 144 and 148 pounds, which is my goal weight. My daily intake is between 1100 and 1300 calories.

Keep in mind, you should discuss with your physician any changes to your diet, especially if your physician has you on a special regimen.

Back in the day, a well-known program counted calories. That same program later changed to a plan where food was divided into breads, proteins, fruits, etc. And you were allotted so many bread foods, protein foods, and so on through the day. (Another form of calorie counting, by the way.) I remember thinking, "I don't want to count everything I eat." Today, they count points. Points are easier to count than calories, it's true. However, counting is still counting. You're going to have to do portion control on some foods in some form. And most of the time, keeping track or counting one thing or another is generally involved. Every product on the grocery store shelves has portion information on the label for your convenience. (By the way, somebody had to count those numbers, so, obviously they must be important.)

There are only two options, make progress or make excuses!

I invested time Googling how many calories are in this and how many carbs in that. With today's technology it's quite simple to find these answers for your needs.

I think I just may have discouraged you. Does it sound like a lot of work? Well, it's not. As you Google, searching out your numbers, be it calories or carbs, write them down. In a few weeks you'll have all your information. Think of the payoff after you gather your basic information on the foods you like to eat.

The result of your search will be eating the things that you like as the scale diminishes in numbers.

This visual guide may help:

1 cup = Size of cupped fist
1 ounce = meaty part of your thumb
1 tablespoon = your thumb minus the meaty part
1 teaspoon = tip of your index finger
3 or 4 oz. of meat, fish or poultry = the size of the palm of your hand.

We enjoy our sweets and our pasta, and my husband absolutely loves steak… any kind of steak (cholesterol alert). I can't tell you how awesome it is not to feel deprived. The time spent researching what I needed to do to modify the meals that we desired was the price for such incredible freedom.

Do you have a scale in the house? I have two scales. I have the dreaded bathroom scale, and I have a little digital kitchen scale. They both take seconds. When I began this journey 2 years ago, I used my little kitchen scale every day. I weighed meats and pasta. (I still use my kitchen scale occasionally, but now, most of the time, I can judge proper amounts.) And as a result, my kitchen scale took the "ugh" out of the bathroom scale. Please note that a scale is just another tool for the accountability which some of us are in need of.

I have found for most meals, whether it be breakfast, lunch, or dinner, that I'm always a little off on something like the carbs or the sodium. This is alright because at the end of the day, it all equals out to where they should be.

Steve's thought: "I can't believe it's not a diet, diet book!

Chapter 7 -- *What About Carbs?*

Let's look at good carbs and bad carbs. This next section will help you determine what carbs you prefer to consume and hopefully help you have a better understanding of why the word "carbohydrates" has such a bad rap. This is also one of those areas where some carbohydrates require modification. It's that simple.

As you search out the food for your new diet, you will see on the labels just some of the following: natural sugar, no sugar added, low calorie sweeteners, sugar alcohols, reduced calorie sweeteners, complex carbohydrates, simple carbohydrates, processed grains, refined grains, whole grains, and a litany of more of the same. It is a wonder that any regular person can find a diet while trying to sort through this encyclopedia of food labels.

The simple thinking for today is that foods are either good or bad. Do you eat it, or do you avoid it? What is the truth?

Carbohydrates can be healthful or harmful, depending on the carbohydrate and how much of it you eat. It is true that it's very easy to eat too much of them. So, it is logical that it is easier for many dieters to just cut them out completely Eating carbohydrates in moderation will do you no harm. Over consumption of anything is were problems occur.

Nothing is wrong with carbohydrates. Highly processed grains and added sugars are not the best things to consume, not because they are carbohydrates but because, for the most part, they have been robbed of nutrients. They raise insulin levels and they are often high in unhealthy fats and sodium, not to mention some weird ingredients that we can't even pronounce. But carbohydrates are not evil. It is junk food that is evil.

There are always new studies coming out about carbohydrates. All of these "new studies" can cause decisions for healthier eating and weight loss to be very confusing. Shedding those extra pounds is not entirely about carbohydrates, as some may lay claim. Because some types of carbohydrates are better for your health than others, being informed will help you make better choices.

Mayoclinic.com recommends buying fresh, frozen and canned fruits and vegetables without added sugar instead of fruit juices and dried fruits, which have more calories. Also, opt for whole grains over refined grains, which are stripped of the parts of the grain that contain their nutrients.

Stick to low-fat dairy products to reduce saturated fat and calories. Limit the intake of foods with added sugars.

Read your labels!

Let's start with complex and simple carbohydrates.

COMPLEX CARBS

These are the preferred carbohydrates. Complex carbohydrates are the ones that give your body the best fuel. They break down more slowly, giving you steady blood levels throughout the day. As a result, you feel less hungry and irritable when afternoon rolls around.

Most good carbohydrates are low to moderate in calorie content, so you can eat filling amounts and satisfy your hunger without going overboard. They are devoid of refined sugars and refined grains which is directly linked to our current epidemic of obesity and Type II diabetes. They are low in sodium and saturated fats. They are also very low or almost zero in cholesterol and contain no trans fats. Complex carbs include:

    Fresh Fruits

Non-starchy Vegetables
Whole Grains
Nuts and Legumes
Dairy Products not sweetened with sugar

A point of interest here... one of my past diet plans suggested that the best time to consume fruit was on an empty stomach.

There are some websites that suggest this theory and there are those that say it is a myth. But it seems to me that most of them do agree that eating fruit on an empty stomach aids in weight loss and is a healthier option for the diabetic.

Since obesity and diabetes run rampant in our country, and although fruit is good for you any time of day, you should choose for yourself when it is best for you. Think about looking into this.

As that past diet plan had recommended, I would suggest that you enjoy fruits an hour before or two hours after a meal. I believe this will also aid in lowering caloric accumulation. I personally count fruits as a free food *"when"* I eat them on an empty stomach and generally don't add their caloric value to my daily intake number.

I feel that because this theory is suggested for the obese and the diabetic and so it is a sound practice for others to consider.

SIMPLE CARBS

Your body quickly breaks down these carbohydrates, spiking your blood sugar, and you will find yourself looking for a snack very shortly after your last meal.

Most of your processed bad carbohydrates are high in caloric density and refined sugars. They are high in refined grains and low in or devoid of nutrients and fiber. They are often high in sodium. They are also sometimes found to be high in saturated fat, cholesterol, and trans fats. Simple cabs include:

> Refined grains like white bread and white rice
> Processed foods -- candies, cake, cookies and chips
> White potatoes
> Sweetened drinks
> Sugar

A point of interest here... cookies, cakes, and even candy and chips can be made with no or little processed food in them. There are some delicious sweet tooth ideas in the recipe section of this book.

Most people have heard the phrase or statement, "good carbs - bad carbs." Where do you go from here? Obviously, you will want to make the majority of your choices from the complex carbohydrates, the good carbs. That does not mean that simple carbohydrates are off the table. The following list is not a list of do's and don'ts. You don't have to cut out enriched pasta and ice cream. I am very aware that many will say, "I don't eat such and such bad carbs because there is no nutritional value." Keep in mind that you can get your nutrients from the rest of your balanced meals throughout the day.

Please be aware that this is only carbohydrate information and a simple guide. Some of the good carbohydrates are not calorie friendly.

Again, read your labels. Stay away from carbohydrates made in factories or laboratories that are OVERLY processed and stripped of fiber, nutrients, and water, and then filled with added fats, salt, and sugars. These products become unrecognizable as a food. Read your labels.

And of course, I follow my mom's wise advice, "Eat everything in moderation." My beautiful, pasta eating mom is 92 years young as I put these words on these pages. She has lived her entire adult life weighing between 130 and 150 pounds.

The following pages contain a general list of good carbs and bad carbs for your review. You may see some of the bad carbs in some of my recipes in the recipe chapter. Remember the key phrase "moderate and modify."

> *Be faithful in the small things because it is in them that your strength lies.*
> *Mother Theresa*

Good Carbs, Bad Carbs

Vegetables

Good Carbs

Dark leafy greens (all types, such as spinach, kale, lettuce, arugula, purslane and bok choy)

Onions

Peas

Mushrooms

Asparagus

Artichokes

Peppers (all types)

Cauliflower

Broccoli

Jicama

Celery

Eggplant

Cabbage

Brussel Sprouts

Green Beans

Garlic

Fennel

Radish

Sea vegetables such as wakame and dulse

Cucumber

Zucchini

Summer Squash

Pumpkin

Sweet Potato *

Root vegetables such as carrots and parsnips

Winter squash such as acorn *

Tomatoes

Bad Carbs

White Potatoes

Fruits

Good Carbs

Berries, such as blueberries, acai, strawberries, and blackberries

Melons such as honeydew and cantaloupe
Tropical fruits such as pineapple, mango, and papaya *
Kiwi *
Tree fruits such as apples and pears
Citrus fruits such as oranges, * lemons and limes
Grapes
Stone fruits such as cherries, peaches, apricots, and plums

Bad Carbs

Dried fruits such as raisins and prunes

Fruit juices
Fruit leather

Grains/Grain Products

Good Carbs

Quinoa
Whole wheat products
Brown rice
Amaranth
Millet
Sprouted grains
Whole oats

Wheat germ
Bran
Whole grain or sprouted grain bread products

Whole grain pasta
Low-carb pasta

Bad Carbs

White rice
White flour
White bread
Breakfast cereal
Quick oats
Couscous
Pasta
Baked goods (like donuts, cake & muffins)

Corn
Cream of Wheat

Nuts/Seeds

Good Carbs

Almonds

Walnuts

Pecans

Brazil nuts
Pine nuts
Chia seeds
Sunflower seeds
Macadamia nuts
Flaxseed
Pumpkin seeds
Unsweetened nut butter
Hazelnuts
Tahini

Bad Carbs

Corn nuts
Honey roasted nuts
Nuts with a seed or
Sweetened nut butters

Legumes

Good Carbs

Peanuts
Cashews
Soybeans

Kidney beans *
Lima beans *
Fava beans *
Adzuki beans *
Peas *
Pinto beans *
Black beans *
Chickpeas *

Bad Carbs

Sweetened peanut or cashew butter

Dairy Products

Good Carbs

Whole milk *

Cream Cheese

Unsweetened yogurt
Sour cream
Butter

Bad Carbs

Ice cream
Sweetened yogurt
Skim, 1% and 2% milk

Snacks

Good Carbs

Pickles
Olives
Whole grain crackers *

Bad Carbs

Potato chips
Pretzels
Corn chips
Popcorn
Candy
Cookies
Rice cakes
Crackers
Granola bars

Condiments

Good Carbs

Mustard (unsweetened)
Mayonnaise
Pickle relish (not sweet)
Vinegar
Oil and vinegar salad dressing
Full fat creamy salad dressing, such as ranch
Sriracha

Bad Carbs

Low fat salad dressing
Ketchup
Honey mustard
Barbecue sauce

Sweeteners

Good Carbs

Stevia
Aspartame **
Sucralose **
Agave nectar

Bad Carbs

Refined sugar (white or brown)
Corn syrup
Honey
Maple syrup

Beverages

Good Carbs

Water
Coffee
Tea

Diet soda **
Dry wines

Hard liquor

Bad Carbs

Soda
Juice
Sweet tea
Sweetened beverages
Sweet wine
Drink mixers (containing sugars)

*   **Denotes higher glycemic food - eat in moderation**
** **Contains chemicals that may be harmful**

Chapter 8 -- *Darned Processed Foods*

I want to address processed foods. I use them. The major problem with processed foods is when they are eaten in excess.

Let's look at sugar. I'm certainly not trying to say that it's good for you. It's not, but I have to go with my mom on this one. It's all about moderation. Read your labels. Most things in excess are not healthy. Again, it's about choosing what you're okay with and what's going to work for you to drop that weight. My husband and I don't use white cane sugar. But I do use white flour in a few of my recipes. Choices!

Please don't misunderstand me. I am not an advocate of processed foods. In my search for our diet, I came across several articles promoting the healthy and a sister article proclaiming the harmful attributes of almost everything you can mention. There is always a healthier way of whatever path you take. And there is an army of folks that are willing to tell the better way.

I'd like to take a side track of this journey here. It may explain some of my choices and help you make yours.

My husband and I live on a 44-foot sailboat. Her name is Imagine. It's a lifestyle of few. We both feel so fortunate to be living our dream.

My mom was raised on a produce farm. So I grew up on fresh foods. Personally, it would be easy for me to go green and clean on everything. They are all foods I enjoy. But in all practicality, it would be impossible to provision my galley aboard Imagine with fresh fruits and veggies with any consistency. Our lifestyle dictates that sometimes I have to provision my food pantry for 2 weeks, maybe 3, before I can get to a store to replenish our provisions. For this reason, I had to find choices that work for us.

You will also notice that I use a lot of shortcuts. For example, I start my chicken soup with a prepared chicken broth. You'll see that my quick lasagna-ziti recipe "Zitiagna" is amazingly easy. I use a starter sauce for my pasta. Shortcuts and quick meals also came about because of our lifestyle aboard <u>Imagine</u>. Shortcuts preserve our power sources. I know that if we were back in a land home and I had the time, I would enjoy making my sauce and my chicken broth from scratch. But it's just not practical for me now. It's part of our preferred differences.

My point is this. If it takes some processed foods to lower those numbers on the scale, it's okay. You need to decide what is acceptable to you. I think it would be helpful for you to determine the ratio in your diet of processed foods versus fresh food. As I stated before, one of the main problems with processed foods are when they are eaten in excess.

I have found, after talking to others, interviewing, and discussing the basic contents of ***Time to Stop the Battle" (Eating with Freedom)***, that I have often noticed an uncomfortable silence that occurs. I can almost see through their eyes; their brains are on overload because of what they believe or what they know from what they have read or in some cases, studied. A wall of defense starts to build. When I start to inquire about their eating choices, the individual that I'm speaking to at the moment, more often than not, has the answers... has the best plan... knows what is healthier, and sometimes what is healthiest. This is because they have done the research for themselves and found out what their choices are. And it's obvious that they are waiting patiently to tell me about it. The start of a debate about the best course of action is about to begin.

These individuals are not wrong. On the contrary. It's such a wonderful thing to finally find a solution to your food battle. But when they're talking to you, discussing what they found and what worked so very well for them, they are convinced it's going to work the same for you. It's simply just not always the case.

However, I have found that the individuals who are in the Interview Chapter, those who have shared their experience, have been quite open-minded, having an understanding that we are all different. I appreciate each of them for taking the time to share their weight loss stories and beliefs.

Everyone also has different levels of self-control, opinions, and knowledge of nutrition. I'm fully aware that what worked for Steve and I may not work for you, and that's why this book is not about any specific diet. It's about knowing that the weight has to come off because THAT is the number one health issue for you. It's about looking and searching for a healthier way for you. It's about what you can do and what you're not willing to do. Which way will be most successful at lowering the numbers on the scale? It's about your individuality.

Don't wish for it -- work for it.

Chapter 9 -- *Imagine, Boat Life*

A contribution from my husband Steve.

This is just a little break from the dieting information to show you who we are and what we are about. We are regular folks just like everyone else except that we live in a boat.

"If it were up to you, you would sell everything that we have and move on the boat!"

Somewhere around the summer of 2003, we were spending a few days on our boat, something we did often throughout the summer months on Barnegat Bay in New Jersey. Michele made the above statement to me, to which I replied, "I sure would!" and I was serious. Long story short, during the winter of 2004/2005, we had to go to Florida for a business convention. Our friends, who had both just retired, sailed their boat to Florida for their first winter journey. I really didn't have to be at the convention, so it was decided that I would stay on our friends' boat with them for the first 3 or 4 days, and then, after the convention was done, Michele would join us for the remainder of the week.

We had already talked of living on our boat at some time in the future, but that was several years down the road at that time. Michele joined us on our friend's boat at the end of the convention. By the next day, we were making plans. It was a 10-year plan. By the second day that Michele was on the boat, it became a 5-year plan. But by the end of the week, it became a "let's sell the house and everything we own including our business and move on to our boat." That is exactly what we did, and we sailed to Florida in October of that same year.

We have been living aboard since that time, except for a 2-year break while I traveled for work in order to retire in 2017.

We have traveled up and down the East Coast of the United States three times during 2005 and 2006. We are currently sailing our way back up the coast with a final destination of Long Island Sound.

During the two years that I traveled for work to retire, I changed my diet as the result of two trips to the hospital within a week of each other with A-fib. It was scary! I had already had 3 stents placed in my arteries and walking without chest pain became a non-existent event. I couldn't walk more than 100 feet without having to stop and make an excuse in order to let the chest pain subside. The excuse was meant to not alarm Michele of my **new** chest pains. I didn't want another minor or worse heart attack than those I had had in 2008 and again in 2015.

Since retirement and the loss of 50 plus pounds, I can outwalk Michele, and I get no chest pain. I love to walk today. Since retirement and living aboard, my diet (or change in eating habits), has remained essentially the same, and my weight is still around 180 pounds. I still feel great and walking a mile and a half the other day was effortless.

All of this said, it doesn't matter where you live or what your basic lifestyle is, you can get healthier with the weight loss that you are trying to accomplish.

Life on our sailboat is sometimes eventful, but most other times just totally relaxing. Moving back to a land home (or becoming a land-lubber as other cruisers call it), is not an option for us.

Life aboard has been one of the best things we have done as a couple, and we are both on the same sheet of music when it comes to continuing to live on a boat. We have had the opportunity to see things that people traveling in a car or even motor home don't get to see while traveling for their vacations. When was the last time you were able to see Fort Sumter from Charleston Harbor?

The cruising life allows us to meet people from all walks of life, from different places (even other countries), and everybody has a different boat that they choose to live on. With all of these differences, you would think that finding new friends would be somewhat of a challenge. I must tell you that that is so very far from the truth. When we meet other cruisers, the friendship is almost instant. Cruisers rely on each other for everything. We have met people from our first voyage in 2005. We still see them from time to time. We either see them where they live or on the waterway. They are always there to help us if we need it. I wish that land people could have the many opportunities that are afforded us as cruisers.

Our boat is smaller than the average size apartment, but we have everything that we possibly could want. We have two bedrooms (staterooms), two bathrooms (heads), lots of closet space, a living and dining area (saloon), and a fully functional and loaded kitchen (galley). We have a generator for when we want our air conditioning or need to use a large draw electrical appliance. We have solar panels to maintain our batteries. I am currently sitting at our desk, opposite the saloon which contains a 40" HD television with a 1000-watt home theatre system with surround sound: my man-cave on the boat. What more could I ask for? Nothing! Imagine that!

> *Constant effort, not strength or intelligence, is the key to unlocking our potential.*
>
> *Winston Churchill*

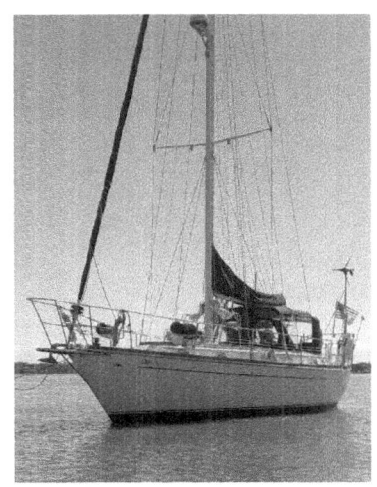

Imagine at anchor.

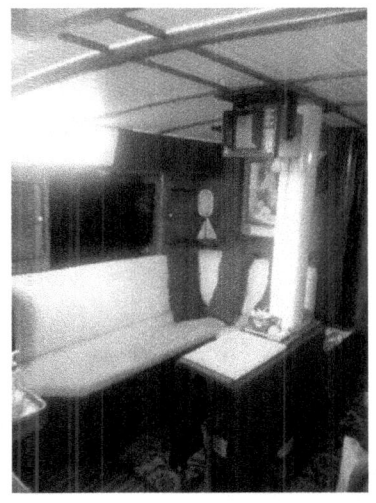

Our Saloon with 40" TV

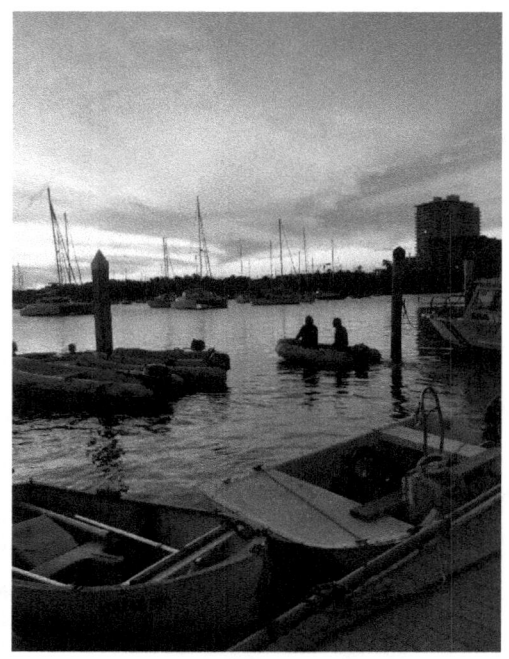

In the dinghy, headed back to our boat at sunset

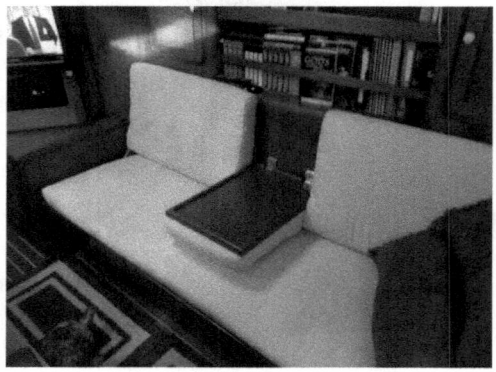

The other side of our saloon.

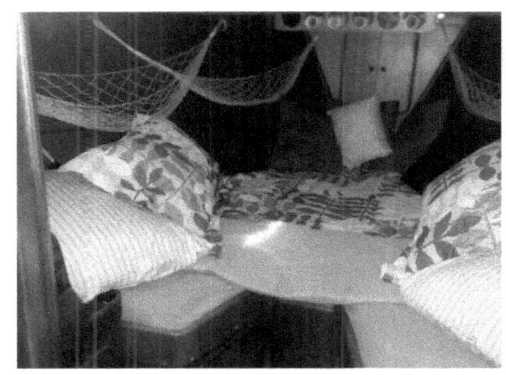

Forward bedroom (V-berth)

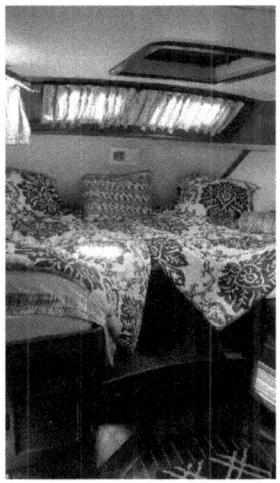

The Captain's Quarters

Steve says, "Seas the day."

Chapter 10 -- *Our Galley*

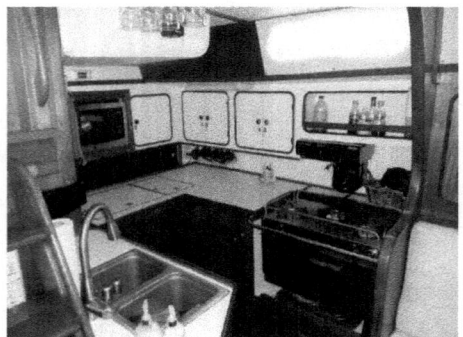

I love my Nu-wave oven, George Foreman grill, Sodastream, and our kitchen scale. I also need to mention that my sister, Patty, gifted to the galley of Imagine, a "non-aerosol oil mister." She ordered it on QVC. I use it every day in so many ways. It is the best gift ever.

Refer to this list when looking at my recipes. This is the list of the main low-calorie processed foods that I use:

- Xtreme Fitness high fiber tortillas
- Nature's Own Life Honey Wheat Bread 40 calories per slice
- Trader Joe beefless ground meat
- Thomas English Muffins high fiber
- Great Value Baking Mix (like Bisquick)
- Thomas Bagel Thins
- Trader Joe Spicy Jalapeno Chicken Sausage Links (or Jennie-O Spicy Sausage)
- Morning Star Farms Hot Sausage Patties
- Morning Star Farms Grillers Original
- Almond Breeze almond milk 30 calories
- Libby Sliced Pineapple Skinny Fruits
- Sliced peaches, no sugar added (any brand)

- PB2 powdered peanut butter
- Splenda
- Stevia
- Jell-O gelatin and pudding no sugar added
- Hunt's Pasta Sauce - Garlic and Herb
- Campbell's Cream soups (98% fat free when I can get them)
- Instant brown rice
- Mrs. Butterworth no sugar added maple syrup
- Smart Balance Light
- Precooked Trader Joe polenta (comes in a tube)

And this is our "we don't drink, we don't smoke" reasoning for the following (not so healthy) food choice. We use either Parkay Spray Butter or I Can't Believe It's Not Butter spray. We love it and if I had to eliminate an unhealthy food from our pantry, this would probably be the first to go. But we are both not willing to part with our spray butter yet.

I do use white flour moderately. We love our ciabatta rolls and our pasta. There are a few more canned foods we use because of practicality such as beans, mushrooms, diced tomatoes, tuna, and clams.

When I fry, I always use a non-stick spray and/or 1 to 2 tablespoons of olive oil and if more liquid is needed, I add chicken broth or water. Chicken broth is one of my "go to" seasonings and overall helpers in my galley.

Chicken broth is an easy purchase but if you would like to make your own, here is an easy recipe for a hearty chicken stock. It's a great chicken soup starter.

Chicken Stock
2 pounds chicken pieces. (wings, backs and thighs)
2 stalks of celery, largely chopped
1 medium onion, largely chopped
2 carrots, largely chopped
4 cloves crushed garlic

1 large sprig parsley
6 quarts of water
   Goya Adobo (red cap) seasoning or sea salt
   Pepper to taste

Cook chicken over low heat until pink is gone. Place the rest of the ingredients in the pot with the cooked chicken. Simmer for 3 hours. Cool and strain. Discard vegetables and chicken as they have no nutritional value. Refrigerate overnight. Skim the fat off the top the next day. (To have homemade stock in your kitchen for future use, you can freeze in quart sized containers.)

MORE LOW-CALORIE FOODS TO CONSIDER

   Our choice for cheeses are fat-free or low-fat. Consider these low-fat or no-fat cheeses: American, cheddar, cottage cheese, feta, mozzarella, parmesan, provolone, ricotta, string. I also use more egg whites than whole eggs and I always have some low-calorie yogurt in the galley fridge.

SOMETHING ELSE TO CONSIDER
"Fat-Free Verses Regular Whole Milk Cheese"

   Most regular whole milk cheeses are not only high in fat but also in cholesterol.

   Major benefit of low-fat cheeses - they do not contain any fat or cholesterol. However, manufacturers often add other ingredients to fat-free Cheese's for taste. One added ingredient is sodium.

> *The best teachers are those who show you where to look but don't tell you what to see.*

The Daily Plate website shows 1/4 cup of whole cheese has 180 mg of sodium, while 1/4 cup of fat-free cheese has 280 mg of sodium. Watch for this if sodium is a concern for you.

The American Heart Association recommends fat-free and low-fat cheeses in your daily diet.

These are some of the veggies that reside in our galley from time to time. I'd like to add that I rarely count calories on my green veggies. For the most part, I view them as a type of free food.

Artichokes
Asparagus
Broccoli
Broccolini
Broccoli rabe
Cabbage
Cauliflower
Celery
Collard greens
Cucumbers
Tomatoes
Zucchini
Dark leafy greens, like spinach, kale, arugula, bok-choy, etc.
Lettuce, all varieties
Mushrooms, all varieties
Snow peas
Sugar snap peas
Green beans
Brussel sprouts
Onions
Peppers, all types

Of course, there is a longer list of veggies available. This is just our regular list of green veggie choices. And yes, I know mushrooms are not green. Actually, they are a fungus, and a healthy fungus at that.

We eat lots of veggies. Steve has mentioned more times than I can count, "I would never have eaten this before." When he says this, he is referring to the mound of veggies on his plate. By the way, along with those delicious veggies at dinner, we always look forward to our side salad; tomato and cucumber with Balsamic Vinaigrette being our favorite.

Veggies are a weight loss key to many diet plans and are needed for a balanced diet. If you are not a fan, I would suggest you start with just one veggie that you enjoy. It will open the door to others that have a like taste. Once you open yourself to one, other veggies will walk right through that door, to your surprise, ready to fill your tummy. That's what happened in our home.

NOTE....Veggies are a great "fill me up" food and a salad with every dinner will help curb your appetite.

Ketchup was used as a medicine in the 1930's!
Really? Really!

Chapter 11 -- *Recipes*

In the following pages you'll find the foods Steve and I enjoy. I have to let you know that Steve was a real trooper as I learned to modify our own eating habits. It was a fun, and sometimes it was a 'too funny taste test adventure" to say the least.

Please remember that I cook using a skillet on a gas cooktop, a Nu-Wave Oven, a George Foreman Grill and an 1100-watt Microwave. Your cooking times may vary slightly from mine. Refer to Pages 52 and 53 to see the specific low calorie processed foods that I use in the following recipes.

BREAKFAST CHOICES IN OUR HOME

A CHAT ABOUT OUR "KEEPING IT SIMPLE " BREAKFASTS...

I want to let you know what's real in our daily diet. These recipes are just some of the dishes that we enjoy. That's what I want to give you, a view of what we actually eat. Reality check… at least my reality, I don't always have the time to spend following recipes, and sometimes the "want to" is just missing. So, although I love to spend time in my galley, preparing meals, I do look for quick, easy and simple meals for those times when the "want to" is "out to lunch."

We aren't cereal eaters. Most of them are loaded with sugar. Personally, I stay away from them because it takes mega servings to satisfy me. Cereal is a weak spot for me. So, I will only purchase a box of cereal with a low sugar content on occasion.

Keeping it Simple and Light in Calories.

Toasted Ciabatta Roll
One of our regulars is simply a toasted ciabatta roll at **200 calories per roll**. It's quick, easy, heartier and more satisfying than a few pieces of toast for my husband. We top them with Parkay Spray Butter. You can also top them with Sugar-Free Jelly if you want something sweet. Our favorite is Apricot.

Toast-Fingers with Syrup
I sometimes drizzle a little Mrs. Butterworth's Sugar-Free Syrup over **toast fingers**. Bread, toasted and cut into finger size sections…"toast fingers".
Approximately 60 calories per slice of bread

Oatmeal
Oatmeal is another one of those personal taste go-to breakfast meals. As a child, I enjoyed, layered in my bowl, 4 saltines; then a serving of oatmeal, dabs of butter, and a sprinkle of sugar and finished off with about 3/4 of a cup of milk. (Still a yum for me.) But today, as boring as it sounds, I like it plain... just cooked in water. **Approximately 150 calories.** Steve eats 1-1/2 servings and likes his with a heaping tablespoon of raisins, Splenda to taste, topped with Parkay Spray Butter.
Approximately 265 calories

Moms Smashed Banana 'n Peanut Butter Muffin
One of my mom's favorite breakfasts is a toasted English Muffin with 2 tablespoons peanut butter, topped with a smashed banana. No PB2 for my mom. She's all about the real deal, crunchy peanut butter.

Approximately 420 calories per serving.

Pancakes with Sausage Links

1-1/2 servings of pancake mix
2 Jimmy Dean Turkey Sausage Links
  Sugar-free maple syrup

Ok... truth... I purchase pre-made pancake mixes and just add water. (Don't forget, read labels to know what you are purchasing.) I don't add the egg, oil or milk. And I generally don't buy the " just add water" premixes.

I always serve 1-1/2 servings for each person. (Use the serving size on the directions for the amount of mix to use). I blend the mix with an equal amount of water then let it rest for a minute. Each pancake is a little less than 1/4 cup of batter. (Makes 3 pancakes.)

Cook them on a griddle or in a frying pan till golden on both sides using a non-stick spray. Top with Mrs. Butterworth's Sugar-Free Syrup (or sugar-free syrup of your choice). Serve with 2 Jimmy Dean Turkey Sausage Links. My husband's favorite breakfast, by the way.

Approximately 300 calories per serving

I'm sorry Fruit Loops lovers... but no matter the color, they all taste the same!

Our pancake sandwich may sound somewhat strange, but I urge you to try it. I think you will be pleasantly surprised.

Pancake Sandwich

1/3 cup pancake mix

1/3 cup water

1 egg

2 Jimmy Dean Turkey Sausage Links

Combine pancake mix and water and let rest for 1 minute. Cook two pancakes on a griddle or in a frying pan using a nonstick spray till golden brown on both sides. Set them aside.

In the same skillet, heat your sausage links and fry up an over easy egg.

Time to serve.... Place your "over easy" cooked egg in-between your pancakes. Add your sausage links to the plate and top it with a serving of sugar-free syrup.

Serves 1

Approximately 340 per serving

Apples come from the same family as roses! Huh!

Omelets

2 egg whites
1 serving of an egg substitute
1 Jimmy Dean Turkey Sausage Link
1/4 cup cooked greens (spinach, broccoli, etc.)
2 ounces reduced fat shredded cheddar cheese
2 tablespoons canned mushrooms, chopped
  Served with 2 slices of toast, 40 calories per slice bread

In a bowl, whip egg white and egg substitute with a fork. Add chopped sausage, mushrooms and cooked greens and stir to combine.

Pour into a non-stick sprayed frying pan. Cover and cook on low heat. When egg mixture is cooked to a soft solid state (partially set), sprinkle some of the shredded cheese, fold in half and top with desired amount of the remaining cheese.

Approximately 280 calories per serving

Bon Appetit!

(Ham and cheese is yum...Also try Feta cheese and spinach. Create your own tastes with the egg mixture...it's a safe breakfast calorically. (I sometimes use Egg-Beaters Southwestern Style. I always choose low fat, reduced fat or fat free cheeses to minimize the cholesterol.)

My Mom says, "A little bit won't hurt you."

Breakfast Burritos

1 serving Egg Beaters Southwestern Style

1 egg white

1 Jimmy Dean Turkey Sausage Link

2 tablespoons reduced fat shredded cheddar cheese

1 Extreme Wellness Tortilla*

Dice sausage. Heat over medium heat. Set aside.

Whisk Egg Beater and egg white together. Cook over medium heat until fluffy. Set aside.

Layer the cooked egg mixture, sausage and cheese in the tortilla. Roll up and enjoy.

There are tortilla roll ups and wraps in the up-coming recipes. If you would like help folding a tortilla so the yum doesn't escape from the bottom on the first bite, visit Google. Search for "instructions on folding a tortilla." It's a helpful find.

Approximately 190 Calories per Burrito

Sausage, Egg 'N Cheese

(On a toasted bagel thin or toasted English Muffin)

One of our favorites, and it's only a 3-minute breakfast. I use a microwave omelet dish.

- **1 Thomas English Muffin or Bagel Thin, toasted**
- **1 egg white**
- **2 tablespoon egg substitute**
- **1 slice fat-free or reduced fat cheese of choice**
- **1 Morning Star Farm Sausage Patty**

Whisk egg white and egg substitute. Pour egg mix into microwave omelet dish. Close dish and place sausage patty on top of dish. Microwave for 1-1/2 minutes while your bagel or muffin is toasting. Layer your sausage, egg and cheese in your bagel or muffin and voila! Can also be done quickly on your stovetop.

Approximately 250 calories using fat free cheese.

We choose to keep our breakfast meals simple and low calorie, keeping them below 350 calories. We eat most of our calories after 6-pm with dinner and our evening snacks.

> *The best thing about the future it that it comes only one day at a time!*
>
> *Abraham Lincoln*

TIME TO ADDRESS LUNCHES

Oh-my-goodness, reality check again! At least it's the reality I have observed and have in common with most of my friends and family. I believe it to be real for the greater majority as well. I guess if you have a cook in the kitchen at all times, you can have anything you want for lunch. But in *my* reality, as I have experienced, lunch is in the middle of the day. It's break time. It's a time to eat. But what about the time before lunch? What are you doing? In my world, prior to lunch, I am just busy. The day, and time in my life of course, determines what kind of busy I am. In my young adult years, I was busy with my babies. Plus, I was a working mother with a full-time job. So, needless to say, some of those Mommy days I was working, and lunch was break time. As my children got older, I continued to work, and lunch continued to be my break time. Today I am fortunate and blessed to enjoy retirement. But guess what…aboard our home, sailing vessel <u>Imagine</u>, I find myself very busy again which, by the way, I see as a very good thing. Still, lunch is break time. Morning is a time for cleaning and preparing for the rest of my day. It is essential to get accomplished as much as needed prior to the heat of the day. Once again, a short preparation time for lunch.

I am emphasizing the fact that lunch is generally a break time because it's not a part of the day that is spent in preparation of mid-day eating. For most, I believe, it is that part of the day to stop.... eat....and gather yourself for your agenda for the rest of the day. This of course is not always the case, but I have experienced it to be the norm most days. I have included this topic in the questionnaire. Those who were interviewed may have different experiences. For many, it's a "grab and go" time of day.

Because we are big night time snackers, my goal is always to keep lunch as light as I can calorically as well.

With that being said, the following are some of our afternoon eats.

LUNCHES

Lunch time is generally when we enjoy our Veggie Sticks as a side, and a dessert always follows. Jell-O, with a large dollop of whipped cream or ice-cold peaches (either canned or fresh), is our norm and very refreshing. It is the making for a happy sweet tooth. We try to keep our lunch desserts under 150 calories.

In the following lunch time suggestions, I always use low calorie bread (40 to 45 calories per slice). And when you see a cheese in any recipe, it will always be fat-free or reduced fat. I use Miracle Whip Light and 96% lean ground beef.

Here is a simple start.......

Ham 'n Cheddar Cheese
Turkey 'n Swiss Cheese

5 slices ham or turkey breast

1 slice cheese of choice

   Mayo or mustard (Steve loves horseradish mustard)

2 slices 45 calorie bread,

2 or 3 slices of tomato (optional)

   Lettuce leaves (optional)

Serves 1

Approximately 280 calories

Add a serving of veggie sticks and peaches, for another 175 calories

> *The ultimate measure of a man or a woman is not where he or she stands in the moment of comfort and convenience, but where he or she stands at the time of challenge and controversy.*
>
>   *Rev. Martin Luther King*

Toasty Ham 'n Cheese Melt

2 slices bread, toasted, 45 calories per slice
4 slices of ham
2 ounces reduced fat sharp cheddar cheese
1 tablespoon Miracle Whip Lite (you can substitute lite mayo)

Heat your 4 slices of ham on a microwave safe dish for 10 seconds. Place 2 oz. of reduced fat shredded sharp cheddar cheese throughout the layers of ham. Microwave for approximately 20 seconds. Spread a light amount of mayo on both pieces of your warm toast. Place your warm ham and cheese on the toast.........time for Yum!

Serves 1
Approximately 340 calories

A nice addition to this melt would be a 1/2 cup of fat free cottage cheese and 8 oz. of icy cold no sugar added peaches mixed together. Add a dollop of whipped cream,

Add another 150 calories

DON'T Sandwich It.....WRAP IT

2 slices of ham or turkey
1 slice of reduced fat cheese of choice
  Extreme Wellness Tortillas
  Tomato slices
  Shredded lettuce
1 tablespoon onion, sliced
  Thinly sliced cucumber
  Miracle Whip Lite to taste

Layer it...Wrap it ...using an Extreme Wellness Tortilla Wrap. Yum, so good! Ohhh, ...serve with pickles and Veggie Sticks of course.

Approximately 230 calories per wrap

How About Hot Diggity Dogs

There are tasty 40 to 60 calorie dogs on the market. You can make them cheesy or Sauerkraut them up, or how about a bit of chili 'n cheese...yum! Think about topping them with diced onions.

Serve with some low-calorie chips or Veggie Sticks and maybe a dill pickle on the side. A sliced fresh farm picked tomato is always a plus.

Plain dog in the bun, approximately   **160 calories**
With reduced fat shredded cheddar   **250 calories**
Above with 2 tablespoons chili   **280 calories**
With dog in the bun and kraut   **165 calories**

Enjoy with a side (1/2 cup) of Baked Beans (next page) and add around 100 calories.

Baked Beans

15 ounce can baked beans
2 tablespoons bacon bits
1 teaspoon Worcestershire Sauce
1 teaspoon horseradish mustard
1 tablespoon + 1 teaspoon ketchup
1 tablespoon + 1 tablespoon Brown Sugar (Page 136)
1 tablespoon onion, minced
1/4 teaspoon molasses
1/8 teaspoon sea salt
1 teaspoon Kitchen Bouquet (optional)

Combine ingredients in a saucepan and simmer for 10 minutes, stirring occasionally.

Makes 4 servings
Approximately 100 calories per serving

You can suffer the pain of change or suffer remaining the way you are.

Joyce Meyer

Wraps

When I want to cut the carbohydrate intake for sandwiches or wraps, I substitute lettuce leaves for the bread products and make a Lettuce Sandwich or a Lettuce Wrap. I use 2 or 3 Romaine leaves, lined, slightly overlapping each other, add the sandwich filling and enjoy. Or, for a crispier wrap, I do the same with Iceberg Lettuce. The following recipes can all be served as Lettuce Wraps. (I put about anything in a lettuce wrap.) Don't forget to use your 50 calorie Xtreme Wellness Tortilla Wraps if you don't want lettuce wraps. There are also 50 and 60 calorie, whole wheat flatbread wraps available.

Cheeseburger Wraps

1/4 pound of 96% lean ground beef

1 slice reduced fat cheese of your choice

   McCormick Grill Mate Hamburger Seasoning to taste

   Tomato slices, (optional)

   Dill pickles, diced (optional)

   Onion slices (optional)

   Ketchup to taste

Season ground meat with McCormick Grill Mate Hamburger Seasoning to taste. Cook like a patty or just cook the loose beef until done. Place patty (or the loose beef), in your wrap of choice, add cheese, sliced tomato, diced dill pickle, onion and ketchup....mmmm!

Approximately 200 calories with a lettuce wrap
Approximately 250 calories with a tortilla
Approximately 320 calories with a 120-calorie hamburger bun

Chicken or Tuna Salad Lettuce Wrap

7 ounce can solid white tuna*
5 ounce can chunk light tuna*
1/2 stalk celery, minced
3 tablespoons onion, minced
1/4 cup Miracle Whip Lite + added for spreading on tortilla
Sea salt and pepper to taste

Mix the above ingredients until well blended and place in a lettuce wrap.

Of course, cheese and tomato is always a nice addition along with a dill pickle on the side.

*You can substitute 12 ounces of chicken for the tuna.

Serves 5
Approximately 88 calories per lettuce wrap
Approximately 138 calories in a tortilla
Approximately 208 calories in a 120-calorie hamburger bun

Egg Salad   Another winner in a lettuce wrap!

5 hardboiled eggs, chilled and chopped (only use two of the yolks)
3 tablespoons celery, minced
2 tablespoons Miracle Whip Lite
1/2 teaspoons mustard
1 tablespoons onion, minced
2 tablespoons dill pickle, minced
   Sea salt and pepper to taste

Mix together until well incorporated. Place in your lettuce wrap.

Serves 2

Approximately 130 calories per serving
Approximately 180 calories in a tortilla
Approximately 215 calories on 40-calorie toast
Approximately 250 calories in a 120-calorie hamburger bun

This is great on open faced toast!

Chicken Fajita Wraps

Great for lunch or dinner!

10 Extreme Wellness Tortillas
1 large onion, sliced largely
1 green bell pepper, sliced into strips
1 pound of chicken breast, sliced into strips
1/2 teaspoon chili powder
1/4 teaspoon Goya Adobo
1/2 teaspoon garlic powder
1 teaspoon dried oregano
1 fresh lime (optional)
2 tablespoon olive oil + olive oil in an oil sprayer
3/4 teaspoon cumin
2 teaspoon Worcestershire Sauce
10 ounce can Ro-Tel Diced Tomatoes with Chile's
1-1/4 cup reduced fat shredded cheddar cheese
   Shredded lettuce

Slice onion and pepper into strips. Place in a non-stick skillet with olive oil and cook over medium heat approximately 7 minutes or until tender. Remove from skillet and set aside.

Slice chicken breast into approximately 1/2" strips, spray same skillet lightly with extra virgin olive oil (EVOO) from your sprayer, add chicken strips, sprinkle with chili powder, cumin, Worcestershire, Goya, garlic powder, and oregano and cook for approximately 10 minutes, or until chicken is done.

Return onion and pepper mix to skillet and add can of Ro-tel diced tomatoes and simmer for an additional 3 minutes.

Spam! What is it?

Place the chicken mix into the wrap and add shredded lettuce and a bit of shredded cheese to each of your wraps, roll up and enjoy.

Optional: Squeeze fresh lime juice into the wrap before rolling.

Makes 10 wraps
Approximately 190 calories per wrap

I'm A PB2 Lover Wrap....

If you love PB2 like I do, this is simple, juicy, crunchy, refreshing and quick.

Cucumber sliced thin, lengthwise
1 tablespoon sugar free jelly
3 or 4 lettuce leaves for wrap
2 tablespoons PB2

Cover cucumber with PB2. Brush some sugar-free jelly in your lettuce leaves. Place coated cucumber in your jelly brushed bed of lettuce wrap and roll it up.

Approximately 80 calories per wrap

I'd like to complete the lettuce and tortilla wraps by encouraging you to use your imagination. Be they lettuce or tortilla, are excellent for leftovers. Think about your leftover meatloaf and mash potatoes, or taco leftovers. And how about leftovers from a casserole or barbeque night? Leftovers from the night before in any form make great "break time" lunches.

AND.........THAT'S A WRAP!

Remind yourself that it's okay to not be perfect.

Burgers Moving on to one of Steve's favorites.

1 Morning Star Farm Griller Original
1 ciabatta roll, toasted
1 slice reduced fat cheese of your choice
   Lettuce leaves
   Sliced Tomato
   Salt, pepper and ketchup to taste
   For variety, you can add 1 tablespoon onion, and dill pickle

I heat the Morning Star Farms Griller in the toaster or cook in a non-stick frying pan. When cooked, layer all the ingredients in the toasted ciabatta roll.

We have found that most of the veggie burgers in the grocery stores cold case are very tasty.

Approximately 380 calories per sandwich. Add 130 calories if served with veggie sticks.

Making this Quarter Pounder with Cheese using 96% lean ground meat is also approximately 380 calories.

You can make this burger with the following if you are watching your cholesterol...but exercise caution with your total sodium intake for the day.

Lower Cholesterol Ground Meat Blend
1/2 lb. 96% Lean Ground Beef, cooked and added to 6 oz. Trader Joe Meatless Ground Beef
COMPARISON CHART

1 Serving (4 ounces):	Cholesterol	Sodium
96% Lean Ground Beef	65mg	76mg
Lower Cholesterol Mix Above	32mg	154mg

Cheeseburger Salad   Now MY favorite burger!

This is exactly what it says it is! I love salads...I love cheeseburgers...why not?

1/4 pound of 96% lean ground beef, cooked
1/3 cup reduced fat cheese of choice (I like American)
1/4 cup onion, diced
  Sliced baby dill pickles
1 large Roma tomato, diced

Now all that is left is the bun and bit of lettuce.
Forget the bun... place your ingredients (cheese and burger fixin's) in a large bowl with your greens of choice, (I like Iceberg and spinach mix), approximately 2 cups.... Don't forget the squirt of ketchup, it's a must. This also works great with cheese steak fixin's.

Serves 1
Approximately 250 calories

Grilled Sausage Sandwich

Lastly another one of our lunch break time meals is a simple fried (with a spray of olive oil; or cooked on our George Foreman grill), spicy chicken sausage (Trader Joe) sandwich in a toasted 6" sub roll. As I mentioned previously, it's important to enjoy the foods that you grew up with. The ones that have a special memory. This is one of them for me.

1 Toasted 6"sub roll

2 Trader Joe Spicy Jalapeno Chicken Sausage Links (Substitute Jennie-O Spicy Chicken Sausage Link if not available)

Heat the sausages in a skillet on the stovetop over medium heat and raise the heat for the last couple of minutes to crisp the casing. Slice sausages length-wise and place on the toasted roll. Enjoy.

Approximately 400 calories per sub (480 with Jennie-O Sausage)

I need to take a side Journey here and tell you about the "special" that accompanies my yummy sausage in a roll. I hope it brings back a heart-felt memory for you.

Although growing up in the city, I spent a lot of time as a child on the farm. It was my Mother's homestead where she was raised with her 9 siblings.

My Mother and her sister Rose were very close. The family's farm became the home of my Uncle Freddy, Aunt Rosie and close-to-my-heart and best play pal...my cousin Theresa. My weekly plea was, "Mom, pleazzzze, can I spend the night". They were my other family. I vividly remember waking up to the smell of the sausage frying up in the pan. There would be my aunt Rosie, at the stove, with her apron on. As you can see this is a side journey of the heart.

The sausage sandwiches in toasted rolls are very yummy. But more than that, they are a reminder of my loving Aunt Rosie at the stove in her apron...she is missed...

We are all truly connected with our food. It's a big deal. It's something that should not be denied. A lot of our connections are from tradition. But some, like my sausage in a roll, are also of the heart.

Well that's it for mid-day --- lunch time --- Break time foods. Bon Appetit!

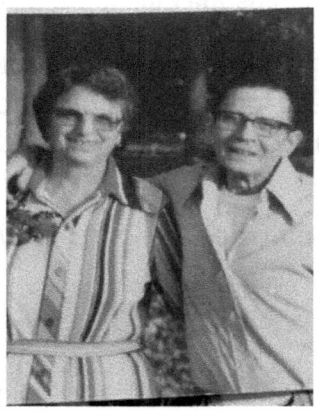

My Aunt Rosie and Uncle Freddy

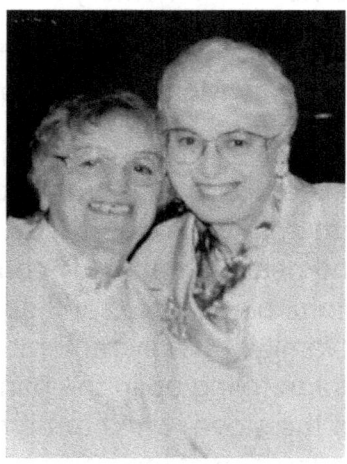

Aunt Rosie and Mom

Me

My Cousin Thresa (Tree)

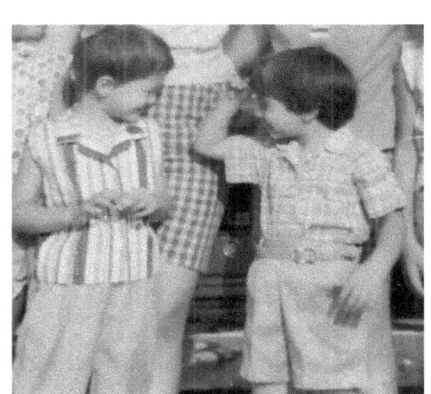

My best play pal...my cousin Theresa

DINNERS

Spagetts With Bolognese Sauce
Bolognese Sauce (One of my galley quickies)

- 16 ounces of marinara or Hunts Herb and Garlic sauce, choice
- 1 pound of lean ground beef, (I use blend on Page 77)
- 4 ounce can mushroom pieces
- 1/8 cup grated parmesan cheese
- 1 tablespoon fresh basil, chopped
  - Pepper to taste
- 1/4 Tsp Goya Adobo

Brown ground meat. (I cook the 96% beef then add the Trader Joe meatless ground beef with the other ingredients.) Add the rest of the ingredients, stir and simmer for 10 minutes.

Spagetts

- 1lb. pasta of choice, (I prefer linguine or fettuccine)
  - Parmesan to taste

Cook pasta until al dente. Add Bolognese sauce to your pasta. Mix and serve with grated parmesan cheese.

For a spicy, hot, kick to this dinner, add a few drops of G-Moms' Pepper Sauce (Page 117)

Serves 4
Approximately 620 calories per serving

I like to spice this dinner up, so I cook up a Trader Joe's Jalapeno Chicken Sausage Link and serve a small salad per person with this meal, which will add 150 to 200 calories per serving.

A Squashy Alternative Spagetts

Make the previous recipe but substitute either spaghetti squash or Zucchini noodles. There are times when I have prepared this meal with half pasta and half zucchini noodles or spaghetti squash. This is a very low carb meal.

Approximately 200 calories per serving

Cooking Spaghetti Squash

Pierce 3 or 4 times in different places with a steak knife and microwave approximately 5 minutes or until soft. Cut squash in half lengthwise. Scoop out and discard seeds. (At this time, you can choose to season or wait until it's completely cooked. I always season mine after I scrape the strands out of the shell.)
Place halves on a microwave safe dish.... cut side down in about 1/4 cup of water. Microwave an additional 7 minutes or until skin is soft and can be pierced with a fork. Your squash is cooked and ready to be spaghetti-fied. Use a fork to scrape out strands. Voila....spaghetti

Apply the same instructions for baking. Instead of returning them to the microwave for 7 minutes, place halves cut side down in a large baking dish. Bake at 400 for 30 minutes using a half a cup of water.

Don't wait for opportunity. Create it!

Zucchini Noodles

Making zucchini noodles with a handheld Veggetti Shredder is like sharpening a pencil back-in-the-day.

Cut stalk connecting end of the zucchini off. Place that end in the shredder and twist. Voila...there's your noodles. I use my kitchen scissors to cut them shorter. Next, you fry and dry.

FRY -- In a large non-stick frying pan, place your zucchini noodles along with a tablespoon of olive oil. Toss them on high heat until they are hot in temperature for approximately one minute or two. Your goal is not to cook them necessarily but to get them hot in temperature. The 'noodle' texture will be lost if overcooked.

DRY -- Immediately, remove them and squeeze them dry between either paper towels or a cheesecloth. (3 medium size zucchinis are about 2 to 3 servings.)

Time to top with your Bolognese sauce. (Previous recipe.)

Amount of servings depends on the size of your spaghetti squash. And don't worry! Calorically, you can feast on this and the zucchini noodles all day long.

Compare 2 cups of pasta weighing in at 480 calories and 90 grams of carbohydrates.

AND

Two cups of zucchini noodles at 66 calories and 12 grams of carbohydrates.

AND

Two cups of spaghetti squash noodles at 80 calories and 14 grams of carbohydrates.

Hearty Escarole Soup

Bite Size Meatballs (Make ahead of time)

1 pound of 96% lean ground beef
1/3 cup bread crumbs
1/3 cup parmesan cheese
1 egg
1/4 cup almond milk, 30-calorie
1/4 teaspoon oregano

Mix and shape into bite sized balls. Place in non-stick pan and bake in the oven at 350 for 15 minutes with 1/4 cup of water. Or cook in a skillet on stove top over medium/low heat. Set aside cooked meatballs.

Now We're Ready to Make the Soup!

Meatballs (above)
1 pound of chicken breast
1 stalk celery, diced
1/2 small onion, chopped
1 clove garlic, minced
1 head escarole, core removed
3/4 cup of whole kernel corn
2-1/2 quarts chicken broth
1/4 cup Parmesan cheese + additional for optional topping

In a 4-quart pot, sauté garlic, onion and celery in olive oil. Add chicken seasoned with black pepper and sear. Add broth and continue cooking until chicken is cooked through. Remove chicken from the broth, cool and pull apart with a fork into bite sized pieces and set aside.

In a separate pot, boil escarole leaves until tender, about 4 minutes. Don't overcook. Drain and chop escarole.

Add parmesan cheese, chicken and corn to the broth in the pot and stir. Add meatballs with liquid and escarole. Stir and reheat if needed and serve. Top with optional parmesan.

Serves 4
Approximately 420 calories per serving.

You can add drops of G-Moms' Pepper Sauce (Page 117) if you want a little tasty heat.

Make the rest of your life the best of your life!

GRILLING IS ALWAYS A TASTY WINNER

Burgers, chicken breast, legs or thighs...hey, slow grill a whole roaster! Just about anything that you can think of eating can be grilled.

Yum...OH-MY-GOODNESS, I'M MAKING MYSELF HUNGRY....peppers and onions.... asparagus... potatoes of all kinds...carrots.

Don't know what to do with squash? Grill it. Don't forget sausage... hot diggity dogs...corn on the cob... ribeye steaks.... pork butt steaks....short ribs... fish steaks.... lobster tail...

The list goes on and on. Grilling almost always lowers the caloric value and sometimes cholesterol. And there is no "almost" about the awesome flavor that accompanies grilling.

If you are not sure about seasoning on the grill, salt, pepper, and in some cases, a smidgen of butter or olive oil in a foil wrapper will do the trick. Let the grill do the rest.

Some of our favorite seasonings for the grill are Montreal Steak or Chicken Seasoning. I almost always season with Goya Adobo (red cap). Experiment for your individual taste.

Chicken with Broccoli Casserole
This is one of my go-to's!

- **1 pound of chicken breast**
- **10 ounce can of cream of mushroom soup**
- **6 ounces of mushroom pieces**
- **4 ounces reduced fat shredded cheddar cheese**
- **12 ounces frozen broccoli florets (cooked per package)**
- **1 tablespoon parmesan cheese + parmesan for topping**
- **3/4 teaspoon Goya Adobo seasoning, divided**
- **6 ounces ziti noodles, cooked**
- **1 tablespoon olive oil**
  - **Black pepper to taste**

Season chicken breast with 1/4 teaspoon Goya and black pepper. Sear in olive oil. Add a half of a cup of water and continue cooking on low heat until chicken is completely cooked. (Don't discard liquid.) Pull apart chicken breast with a fork or cut into bite-size pieces.

Place chicken pieces with liquid and the remaining ingredients in a large baking dish. Mix together and bake for 20 minutes at 350 degrees.

You can also place your ingredients in a microwave safe bowl and cook on high for approximately 5 minutes. Top with parmesan to taste, optional.

Serves 2 at approximately 760 calories per serving
Serves 3 at approximately 510 calories per serving

Spinachy Sausage 'N Pasta

3 Trader Joe Jalapeno Chicken Sausage Links
1 cloves garlic, finely minced
2 cups chicken broth
2 tablespoons cornstarch
6 ounces pasta of choice, cooked, (I prefer penne pasta)
1 tablespoon olive oil
10 ounces raw spinach
   Parmesan cheese to taste

Brown minced garlic in olive oil. Slice sausage links into bite sized pieces. Add sausage and simmer over medium heat for 3 to 5 minutes until sausage is heated thoroughly. Add raw spinach and simmer an additional 1 to 2 minutes just until spinach wilts.

Dissolve cornstarch in chicken broth and add mixture to sausage and spinach. Simmer until chicken broth is thickened to a creamy consistency.

Add to cooked pasta in a bowl and toss. Top with parmesan cheese to taste.

Serves 2
Approximately 590 calories per serving

Serve with a side salad.

> *I believe that the greatest gift that you can give to your family and the world is a healthy you.*
> *Joyce Meyer*

Subs Are Great for Dinner

Sausage, Pepper 'N Onion

1 bell pepper, sliced in strips
1 medium onion, sliced in strips
6 ounce can tomato sauce
1/2 pound of Trader Joe Jalapeno Sausage, about 3 links
1 tablespoon olive oil
1 tablespoon parmesan cheese
1/4 teaspoon Goya Adobo seasoning
1/2 teaspoon garlic powder
1 cup chicken broth
1/4 teaspoon G-Moms' Pepper Sauce (page 117)
8 ounces reduced fat shredded mozzarella cheese
  black pepper to taste
  6-inch Sub rolls, toasted lightly

Slice sausage links in bite size pieces, place in pan along with oil. Cook over med heat. Add chicken broth, pepper and onion. Toss frequently until tender, not soft. Add tomato sauce and remaining seasonings except for mozzarella cheese. Simmer for 5 to 10 minutes.

Once in the roll, top with shredded mozzarella cheese.

Serves 4
Approximately 450 calories per serving

Leftover Cheesy Meatballs make a great sub.

2 Cheesy Meatballs (Page 105), cut in half
1 ciabatta roll or roll of choice, toasted
1 tablespoon reduced fat shredded mozzarella cheese

Add meatball halves to the toasted roll with a few tablespoons marinara or Bolognese Sauce (Page 82). Top with shredded Mozzarella Cheese.

Approximately 550 calories per sub

ENJOY! GREAT EATS!

Don't give up because of what someone says. Use that as a motivation to push harder.

Another Low-Cal Sub

4 slices of turkey or ham
2 slices reduced fat cheese of choice
  6-inch sub roll, toasted
  Tomato slices
  Lettuce
  Onion slices

Spritz of wine vinegar, and olive oil. A light sprinkle of oregano is the makings of a yummy Italian flavored sub.

Approximately 420 calories per sub

Try a Pepper Steak Sub…

8 ounces of thinly sliced beef sirloin or round steak
1 bell pepper, slivered
1 medium onion, slivered
  McCormick Montreal Steak Seasoning
1 tablespoon olive oil
1 cup beef broth
1-1/2 teaspoons cornstarch for thickening
4 ounces reduced fat mozzarella cheese, optional
  Black pepper to taste
  6-inch sub rolls, toasted

In a non-stick pan, add oil and cook peppers and onion till tender. Do not overcook. Add steak with McCormick seasoning to taste. Cook until pink (medium to medium rare). Dissolve cornstarch in the beef broth. Add beef broth to above mixture in the pan and simmer for 5 minutes. Add black pepper to taste. Optional: Top each sub with 2 ounces of mozzarella cheese.

(Your carbohydrate portion is in your sub roll, they are filled with protein and a side dish or two of your favorite green veggies makes a nice low-calorie balanced meal.)

Makes 2 servings
Approximately 575 calories per sub

Chicken or Turkey SOS

You don't have to wait for leftover turkey from Thanksgiving to enjoy this delicious meal.

1 pound of chicken or turkey breast
1 tablespoon olive oil
2 cups chicken broth
1-1/2 tablespoon cornstarch
1/3 cup of flour
2 cloves garlic, minced
   Sea salt and pepper to taste
   Sliced 40 calorie bread, toasted

Season breasts with salt and pepper and lightly flour. In a non-stick pan, fry breasts and minced garlic in oil. Remove chicken and allow it to cool enough to handle and shred (pull apart with forks).

Mix corn starch with chicken broth. Return chicken to pan and add broth mixture. Simmer for 5 minutes to a thick gravy consistency.

Toast bread slices
Pour your SOS over toast.

Serves 4
Approximately 320 calories per serving. (With 2 slices of toast (40/45 calories per slice). It's quite safe to have seconds at that calorie count.

A salad and mashed potatoes are a yummy addition to this plate.

You didn't come this far to only come this far!

Cheesy Chicken Fritters
THIS IS A MUST TRY *Thank you, Google!*

1-1/2 pounds of chicken breast

1 whole egg + 1 egg white

1/3 cup Miracle Whip Lite

1/3 cup flour

4 ounces reduced fat shredded mozzarella

2 tablespoon parmesan cheese

1-1/2 tablespoons fresh dill, chopped

   Goya Adobo seasoning or sea salt to taste

   Pepper to taste

Dice chicken. Place diced chicken and remaining ingredients in a bowl and mix. (Not necessary but if time allows, cover and refrigerate for 2 hours.) In a non-stick pan, using a tablespoon, place heaping tablespoon amounts of the mixture and press down to create small patties. Cook over medium heat until brown on both sides.

We enjoy dipping our fritters in light blue cheese dressing.

Serves 3

Approximately 550 calories per serving

Crispy Breading

Prepare each in three bowls:

1/3 cup of flour
2 egg whites, beaten
1/2 cup of breadcrumbs

First dip what you are breading in the flour, then dip in the egg white and finally in the bread crumbs. Cook your breaded item according to its recipe.

Approximately 465 calories total

Shake 'n Bake is a great quickie, but I'm sure that you know that. If this is your choice, shake off the extra breading. Coat the chops lightly.

Spanglish Pork Chops
They are breaded -- but it's ok!

Four 4-ounce boneless pork chops
  Crispy breading (Page 96), or Shake 'n Bake
  olive oil in sprayer
  Medium or hot chunky salsa (your choice)
4 ounces reduced fat shredded cheddar cheese

Crispy bread the pork chops. Place crispy breaded chops in a non-stick oven pan and spray lightly with olive oil. Bake at 400 for 30 minutes. Remove from the oven and generously cover each pork chop with salsa. Top each chop with 1ounce of cheddar cheese. Return to oven and cook until cheese is melted.

Serves 4
Approximately 400 calories per pork chop

Either you run the day, or the day runs you!

Hillbilly Chili

1 pound of 96% lean ground beef

1 medium bell pepper, cubed

1 medium onion, cubed

1 garlic clove, minced

2 stalks celery, chopped

10 ounces fresh mushrooms, chopped

16 ounce can pinto or chili beans

2 tablespoons chili powder

15 ounce can diced tomatoes

1 cup of beef broth

2 tablespoon parmesan cheese

1 teaspoon cumin

1/4 teaspoon oregano

1/2 teaspoon Worcestershire Sauce

   Reduced fat shredded cheddar cheese for topping

Place ground beef in 8-quart pot sprayed with non-stick spray. Add garlic, cumin and chili powder. Stir and brown ground beef.

Stir in broth. Add bell pepper, onion, celery and tomatoes. Cook until veggies are tender. (Tender but not overcooked.)

Add beans and simmer for 5 minutes. Add mushrooms, parmesan cheese and cook for 2 more minutes. Ready to serve. Top with cheddar cheese, also a dollop of sour cream is a great additional topping with or without the cheddar topping.

Serves 3

Approximately 450 calories per serving
For 2 hungry folks approximately 675 calories per serving

Tortilla Soup

1 pound of chicken breast

14 ounce can black beans, undrained

10 ounces frozen corn

1 bell pepper, diced

1 medium onion, diced

3 cloves garlic, minced

1/3 cup celery, chopped

4 cups chicken broth

1 tablespoon extra-virgin olive oil

1 medium carrot, chopped

4 ounces tomato paste

10 ounces cream of mushroom soup

1 tablespoon chili powder

1/2 teaspoon Goya Adobo seasoning (red cap)

1 tablespoon cumin

1/2 tablespoon of fajita seasoning

Dash of red pepper flakes, optional

Splash of mojo juice (you can use lemon juice)

Season chicken with salt and pepper. Sear in heated oil in a 4-quart pot. Add chicken broth and continue to cook until done. When fully cooked, remove chicken and pull apart into bite size pieces with a fork. Set aside.

Dice veggies and combine all remaining ingredients with broth in the 4-quart pot. Cook over medium heat till veggies are tender. Return chicken to the pot.

Serves 4

Approximately 400 calories per serving

Top with reduced fat shredded cheese (optional)

Meatloaf

1 pound of 96% lean ground beef
1/3 cup bread crumbs
1/3 cup parmesan cheese
1 egg
1/4 cup almond milk, 30-calorie
1/4 teaspoon oregano
2 teaspoon fresh basil, chopped
3 tablespoons onion, finely chopped
3 tablespoons celery, finely chopped
2 tablespoons ketchup

Mix and place in a loaf pan or shape into a loaf. Glaze loaf with 2 tablespoons of ketchup and cook at 350 degrees for 20 minutes covered with foil. Remove from the oven and add 1/2 cup of water to bottom and cook another 20 minutes uncovered. Pour drippings in a saucepan and set meatloaf aside.

Gravy

Meatloaf drippings (add 1/2 cup beef broth if drippings are scarce)
1 teaspoon cornstarch
1 teaspoon Smart Balance Light
1/4 teaspoon Goya Adobo (optional)
1 teaspoon Kitchen Bouquet

Cook over medium until thickened. Pour over meatloaf and serve.

Serves 4
Approximately 245 calories per serving

Using the meatloaf recipe, add a few steps and enjoy a delicious.

Shepherd's Pie

Meatloaf ingredients (Page 100)

Gravy ingredients (Page 100)

3 cups cooked instant mashed potatoes

6 ounce can corn, heated

6 ounces frozen mixed vegetables, cooked

Prepare meatloaf mixture and spread evenly in an 8" non-stick backing pan. Follow meatloaf and gravy cooking directions. Set both aside.

Prepare 3 cups of instant mashed potatoes (seasoned with sea salt and butter to taste) to a thick consistency and set aside to cool. Heat corn and set aside. Cook mixed vegetables and set aside.

Spread a thin layer of mashed potatoes over cooked meatloaf mixture in the pan. Spread and press the corn into the first layer of potatoes with your fingertips. Spread another layer of mashed potatoes over the corn. Spread and press the mixed vegetables over the second layer of potatoes with your fingertips. Spread the remaining potatoes over the vegetables like icing on a cake. Place back in the oven for 10 minutes or until vegetables are heated. Pour gravy over the pie and serve.

Serves 4

Approximately 393 calories per serving

> *We know what we are but not what we might be.*
> *William Shakespeare*

Stuffed Cabbage Rolls

Small head of cabbage

3 cups cooked brown rice

4 Trader Joe Jalapeno Chicken Sausage Links

1 pound of chicken breast, cooked

1 tablespoon olive oil

8 cups chicken broth

Salt and pepper to taste

Parmesan cheese sprinkled on top to taste.

Dice sausages into very small pieces and mix with cooked brown rice and set aside.

Place the entire head of cabbage in 8-quart pot of boiling water. Simmer for about 8 minutes. Remove the head very carefully with tongs. Let it cool for a few minutes and start peeling the tender leaves off. Place the head back in the water as necessary to tenderize the remaining leaves. Continue peeling. Set aside separated leaves.

Season chicken with salt and pepper. Sear in olive oil. Add broth and cook until chicken is done. Remove chicken from broth, pull apart into small bite-size pieces and place back in the broth and set aside.

Your meal is now cooked you just need to put it together. Place about 2 heaping tablespoons of the rice/sausage mix in each leaf, roll your leaf closed and place in a baking dish. Repeat until your leaves are filled. Pour your chicken broth mix over your stuffed cabbage to half way up the rolls. Reserve extra broth mix for serving. Bake at 350 for approximately 20 minutes till heated and serve. To serve, place 2 rolls in a soup bowl with about 3/4 cup of broth mix. Top with Parmesan cheese. Makes approximately 16 rolls.

Serves 4

Approximately 500 calories per serving (4 rolls)

30 Minute Low Cal "ZITIAGNE"
(Boat Galley Lasagna)

1/4 pound of 96% lean ground beef, cooked

1/2 cup, about 3 ounces, Trader Joe Meatless Beef

1 cup fat-free cottage cheese

4 ounce can mushroom pieces, drained and chopped

1/4 cup parmesan cheese

4 ounces low-fat mozzarella cheese

1/2 teaspoon Goya seasoning

6 ounces ziti noodles, cooked

1-1/2 cups marinara sauce

Combine ingredients and bake at 350 for 15 minutes or until heated thoroughly -- or -- microwave for 5 minutes until fully heated.

Serves 3
Approximately 550 calories per serving

Believe in yourself and watch yourself doing unbelievable things!

10 Minute Pizza Sauce

I came across this jewel on the internet. It is so delicious!

15 ounces tomato puree

1 teaspoon oregano

1/2 teaspoon dried basil

1/2 teaspoon ground black pepper

1/4 teaspoon salt

1/4 teaspoon Splenda

1/2 teaspoon garlic powder

1/4 teaspoon onion powder

Combine ingredients and simmer for 5 minutes.

THAT'S IT FOR THE SAUCE........

20 Minute Pizza

4 ciabatta rolls cut in half and toasted.

   10 Minute Pizza Sauce (above)

   Toppings of choice

Slice Ciabatta rolls in half and toast. Place toasted halves on non-stick cookie sheet. What do you like on YOUR pizza?

We like ....
A layer of sauce, Turkey pepperoni, Mushrooms, and sausage (Trader Joes), smothered in reduced fat mozzarella cheese.

Broil on bottom rack until cheese melts.... YUM!

Makes 8 servings (8 half ciabatta rolls)
Approximately 185 calories .... varies according to your toppings.

Meatballs....Cheese it up...
Cheesy Meatballs

1 pounds of 96% lean ground beef

1/3 cup bread crumbs

1/3 cup parmesan cheese + parmesan for topping

8 ounces reduced fat mozzarella cheese

1 egg

2 cup marinara sauce or Hunts Garlic and Herb sauce

1/4 cup almond milk, 30-calorie

1/4 teaspoon oregano

Mix and shape into 8 round balls. Use your thumb to create cup like indentation on the top of each while maintaining the meatball's shape. Place in non-stick baking dish and cook at 350 for 25 minutes. Remove from oven, fill the hole that you created with mozzarella cheese and top each meatball with 2 tablespoons of marinara sauce, a dash of oregano and a dash of parmesan cheese and top with mozzarella cheese. Add 1 cup of marinara to the bottom of the pan. Return to oven and bake until cheese is melted, approximately 5 minutes.

Garnish with a basil leaf. The basil leaf is optional, but it's beautiful presentation and adds nice additional flavor.

Serves 4
Approximately 320 calories per serving

Stroganoff

1 pound of 96% lean ground beef

10 ounce can cream of mushroom soup

10 ounce can mushrooms, sliced

1/2 cup light sour cream

2 teaspoons Worcestershire Sauce

2 tablespoons Smart Balance Light

1 tablespoons lemon juice + 1 teaspoon

1 medium onion, chopped

1 teaspoon garlic powder or one large clove finely chopped

1/2 cup beef broth

1 teaspoon Kitchen Bouquet (optional)

   Black pepper to taste

1 pound noodles of choice

Sauté onion, garlic and butter over medium heat. Stir in ground meat and brown. Add soup, mushrooms, Worcestershire, lemon juice, and beef broth. Simmer for 10 minutes. Stir in sour cream until heated. (Do not bring to a boil).

Sprinkle with black pepper, pour over cooked noodles and serve.

Serves 4

Approximately 670 calories per serving

Add a salad of choice and dinner is served.

Braised Country Style Pork Ribs

1-1/2 pounds of country style pork ribs

1 stalk celery, chopped

1 small onion, diced

3 tablespoons Smart Balance Light or olive oil

1 cup chicken or beef broth

1/3 cup flour

   Goya Adobo seasoning to taste

   Black pepper to taste

   Dash of garlic powder

Sauté chopped celery and onion over medium heat with your butter or oil approximately 8 to 10 minutes. Add 1/4 cup of broth as needed to maintain liquid. Remove celery and onion and set aside. Pat ribs dry and season with garlic powder and Goya. Lightly flour. Sear on all sides in the same sauté pan. Place the ribs in a baking pan. Add sautéed vegetable mix and beef broth halfway up the ribs.

Cover and bake 1 hour at 350. Uncover and bake for an additional half hour allowing the liquid to reduce.

Serves 3

Approximately 650 calories per serving

Be somebody that makes somebody feel like something!

Pork Butt Steaks

Lightning speed prep time and so tasty!

2 pork butt steaks, about 1 pound
  Garlic powder to taste
  Montreal Steak Seasoning to taste

Sprinkle seasonings generously on both sides. Press the seasonings in the steaks (both sides) using your fingertips. Bake 25 minutes at 350 degrees covered with foil in a non-stick pan. Flip them and bake for an additional 20 minutes.

Serves 2
Approximately 588 calories per serving

(Also great on the grill)

Easy-Peasy Clam Sauce with Linguine

3 tablespoons Smart Balance Light
1 small onion, diced
2 cloves garlic, minced
  Pinch red pepper flakes
1 tablespoon lemon juice
1 teaspoon oregano
1 teaspoon dry basil
1 tablespoon Old Bay Seasoning
Two 6.5-ounce canned clams with juice
1 teaspoon parsley
1-1/2 teaspoons cornstarch for thickening
1 cup chicken broth
8 ounces linguine, cooked

Whisk cornstarch in the chicken broth with a fork or small whisk. Combine all ingredients except pasta in a pan, bring to a boil, reduce heat and simmer for 10 minutes, stirring occasionally. Serve over cooked linguine.

Of course, a light sprinkle of parmesan won't hurt.

Serves 2
Approximately 610 calories per serving.

There you have it.... boil, simmer and serve.

Polenta Pizza -- One of our favorites.

18 ounces polenta (I use Trader Joe organic pre-cooked)
1/2 cup chicken broth
8 ounces marinara sauce
1 Trader Joe Jalapeno Chicken Sausage Links
4 ounce can mushroom pieces
1/3 pound of 96% lean ground beef
1 cup broccoli florets, cooked*
1/2 cup reduced fat shredded mozzarella
  Parmesan to taste

Combine chicken broth and thinly sliced polenta in a 6-quart pan. Cook over low heat while whisking until blended into a mush.

Steam broccoli florets, chop and set aside. Brown ground beef and set aside. Thinly slice sausage link and set aside. Chop mushroom pieces and set aside.

You're ready to build your pizza. On 2 dinner plates, place half of your polenta mix on each plate and mash it to resemble a round 'pizza crust'.

On each plate ....
Spread approximately 1/3 cup of marinara sauce on top of your polenta pizza crust (mush).

Divide each of the remaining ingredients in half, and layer them over your sauce, finishing with a sprinkle of parmesan and mozzarella.

Place each dish in microwave to heat and you're ready to serve.

Serves 2
Approximately 530 calories per serving

*You can substitute green beans or dices asparagus. Delicious!

Chicken Fingers

1 pound of skinless, boneless, chicken breast
McCormick Montreal Chicken seasoning to taste
Crispy Breading (Page 96)
2 tablespoons olive oil

Cut chicken breast into fingers about the width of a medium carrot and the length of your finger. Place in a bowl and season with McCormick Grill Mates Montreal Chicken seasoning to taste. Remove from bowl and crispy bread the chicken fingers one at a time.

Spray your frying pan with non-stick spray. Place chicken fingers in your heated frying pan with oil and cook on medium heat.

(I have done these in the Nu-wave oven at 350 for 20 minutes and they come out wonderfully crisp. I use my oil sprayer, coating the top to achieve an all-around crispness.)

The simple key to this recipe is a 'light" covering of the flour and bread crumbs.

Serving for 2 at 585 calories per serving
Serving for 3 at 392 calories per serving

We serve them with low calorie blue cheese or ranch dressing. Makes a delicious dip for your fingers!

Sweet 'n Sour Dinner Choices

Sweet 'n Sour Sauce

1 medium bell pepper, largely diced

15 ounce can skinny pineapple chunks

1 small onion, cut in chunks

1/3 cup Splenda

2 tablespoons Worcestershire Sauce

12 to16 ounces chicken stock

1/4 cup wine vinegar

1 teaspoon molasses

1/2 tablespoon ketchup

   Cornstarch for thickening

I like my sauce to be a syrupy consistency. Combine approximately 1 tablespoon cornstarch per cup of liquid. Separate the pineapple from its juice. Set the pineapple chunks aside. Combine the rest of your ingredients along with pineapple juice and simmer for approximately 10 minutes. Add pineapple chunks.

Sauce is a total of 410 calories

Sweet 'n Sour Meatballs

I pour this sauce lavishly over Bite Size Meatballs (Page 85) for Sweet 'n Sour Meatballs.

Serves 4

Approximately 353 calories per serving

Sweet 'n Sour Chicken Fingers

I also use this sauce over bite-size chicken fingers. Just prepare Chicken Fingers (Page 111) and cut in smaller chunks.

Serves 3

Approximately 530 calories per serving

Here is another delicious variation on the Chicken Fingers recipe on Page 111.

Hot Fingers (or Wings)

Chicken Finger recipe (or 1 pound of drumettes)

1/2 cup Louisiana Supreme Chicken Wing Sauce (or Franks Red-hot Wing Sauce)

Sprayer with extra virgin olive oil

Prepare Chicken Finger recipe with cut chicken or drumettes, using the oven method. Place them on a non-stick baking pan, spray a light coating of extra virgin olive oil. I cook these in my Nu-wave oven at 350 for 15 minutes or until lightly crisp.

Remove from the oven and coat the fingers or wings with the sauce of your choice from above. Place back in the oven and continue to cook until the sauce has a glaze appearance, about 5 minutes. Remove and serve with light blue cheese dressing as a dip.

Serves 2

Approximately 585 calories per serving of fingers
Approximately 635 calories per serving drumettes

I believe you will find the taste you are expecting from hot wings with the two sauces that we use. Louisiana Supreme has zero calories and Franks has 5 calories per serving!

Every moment is a fresh beginning!

PORK 'N KRAUT

- 1 pound of boneless pork chops
- 1 medium onion, diced
- 1-1/2 cup chicken broth, divided
- 1 large clove of garlic, minced
- 1 tablespoon olive oil
- 16 ounce can of sauerkraut
  - Garlic powder to taste
  - Black pepper to taste

In a large skillet, sear pork chops seasoned with black pepper and garlic powder in olive oil. Then add 1/2 a cup of chicken broth and simmer for 7 to 10 minutes until there is no pink remaining. Remove pork and cut or break apart pork into bite size pieces. Set aside.

Caramelize onion with minced garlic and a spritz of olive oil in the remaining liquid in pot.

Add sauerkraut, a cup of chicken broth and simmer for 5 minutes. Return your pork to the pot and simmer an additional 5 minutes. Season with black pepper to taste and serve.

Serves 2
Approximately 475 calories per serving

The sweetness of a small baked sweet potato goes nicely with this dish at an added 60 calories.

Zucchini Boats

3 medium to large zucchini
1/4 cup onion, minced
1/2 pound of 96% lean ground beef
1 cup marinara sauce, divided
4 ounce can mushroom, chopped
1/3 teaspoon sea salt
1/2 teaspoon garlic powder
2 tablespoon parmesan cheese + parmesan for topping
1 cup shredded reduced mozzarella cheese, divided

Slice zucchini in half then slice the halves lengthwise and scoop out the center creating a shell. Dice the scooped-out zucchini. Set aside.

Place zucchini shells in a baking dish with 3/4 cup of water. Bake at 350 for 15 minutes. Drain water from baking dish.

Completely brown ground beef with onions, garlic and sea salt. Add diced zucchini centers, 3 tablespoons of marinara sauce and simmer for 7 to 10 minutes. Remove from heat, added mushrooms, 1/4 cup of mozzarella cheese and stir.

Fill your shells (boats), with beef mixture, (approximately 1 heaping tablespoon for each boat). Cover each with the remainder of marinara sauce, place the remainder of mozzarella on boats and top with a sprinkle of grated parmesan cheese. Cook for an additional 5 minutes or until cheese is melted.

Serves 3
Approximately 270 calories per serving

Taco Salad

6 cups of Iceberg lettuce

1/2 pound of 96% lean ground beef

5 ounces hot dog chili

8 ounces refried beans, heated

3 large Roma tomatoes, sliced

3 tablespoons onion, minced

6 ounces reduced fat cheddar cheese

9 tablespoon medium salsa

9 tablespoon fat-free sour cream

Brown ground meat. Add hot dog chili. Combine lettuce, ground meat mix, refried beans, tomatoes and onions. Toss together. Divide mixture into 3 large salad bowls.

Top each serving with 2 ounces of cheese, 3 tablespoons of salsa and 3 tablespoons of sour cream.

Serves 3

Approximately 410 calories per serving

We eat this meal with a serving of veggie straws for an additional 130 calories per serving

> *If you can't fly, then run; if you can't run, then walk; if you can't walk, then crawl, but whatever you do, you have to keep moving forward.*
>
> *Rev. Martin Luther King*

Side Dishes, Sauces 'N Snacks
Let's start the with best first!

G-Moms' Pepper Sauce
If you like teary eyed, nose running hot with crazy yummy flavor, this is it. This is my mother's recipe.

16 ounces vegetable oil (don't use olive oil)

2 tablespoons garlic, minced

3/4 cup red pepper flakes

4 squirts of Tabasco sauce (optional)

Bring oil to a boil. Lower heat to a simmer and add garlic. Cook garlic until golden brown. Add red pepper flakes, stir 30 seconds. Turn stove top off and let it cool. After it cools, drizzle some pepper sauce on a bite of bread and taste to determine if you want to add Tabasco.

Place in a mason jar with a screw lid and keep refrigerated.
Approximately 120 calories per tablespoon

Start easy. Steve uses drops, and I use spoons full of this deliciously hot and tasty sauce.

This sauce is great on:
All pasta dishes! (Including Zucchini and Spaghetti Squash meals)
Hearty Escarole Soup (Page 85)
Spinachy Sausage 'N Pasta (Page 89)
Chicken with Broccoli Casserole (Page 88)
Stuffed Cabbage Rolls (Page 102)
30 Minute Low Cal Zitiagna (Page 103)
Polenta Pizza (Page 110)
Zucchini Boats (Page 115)
and more…

Be creative with this sauce. If you want some added heat with flavor, give it a try.

Buttery Sweet Potatoes

2 medium sweet potatoes, sliced
2 tablespoons Smart Balance Light, melted
1/8 teaspoon cinnamon
1 tablespoon Splenda

Peel and slice sweet potatoes a little more than 1/4 inch thick. Boil until tender. Drain.

Combine Smart Balance, cinnamon, and Splenda. Pour over sweet potato slices, lightly season with sea salt and serve.

Serves 2
Approximately 170 calories per serving

Butternut Nuggets

1 pound of butternut squash, about one large squash, cubed
3/4 cup chicken broth
1 tablespoon Smart Balance Light
1 tablespoon olive oil
  Goya Adobo to taste

It appears like a task but preparing a butternut squash is surprisingly easy. A sharp peeling tool will glide right through eliminating the skin of this delicious squash.

Slice off the stem and the bottom end so that they are both flat. Stand it on its end as you peel. Cut in half lengthwise and scoop out the seeds with a tablespoon.

Lay your halves face down on your cutting board for stability, as you cut them into your desired sized cubes.

In a large skillet, cook butternut squash nuggets in olive oil on low heat for 3 to 4 minutes. Add chicken broth and cook until tender. Broth in the pan should appear velvety. Add small amounts of water if needed as liquid reduces. Before removing from skillet, add Smart Balance and Goya. Toss and serve.

Serves 3
Approximately 135 calories per serving

Cauli Mash

1 head cauliflower cut into florets
1/4 cup parmesan cheese
1 tablespoon fat-free cream cheese
1/4 teaspoon Goya Adobo
1/2 teaspoon garlic powder
1 tablespoon Smart Balance Light

Place cauliflower in just enough water to cover. Cook 8 to 10 minutes or until a fork can easily pierce through the florets. Drain.

Place cooked florets in a blender with remaining ingredients. Blend on high to a mashed potato consistency. Heat in microwave, if necessary, before serving.

Serves 3
Approximately 100 calories per serving

Underground Medley

1 large white potato, cubed
1 large sweet potato, cubed
1 medium onion, largely chopped
1 large or 2 medium carrots, sliced
1 tablespoon Smart Balance Light
1 cup of chicken broth
  Goya seasoning or sea salt

Peel and cube potatoes and carrots. Place butter and cubed veggies in a non-stick pan. Add 1/2 cup of chicken broth. Cook over medium heat for approximately 4 minutes. Add onion and Goya or salt to taste. Add remainder of chicken broth and cook until veggies are tender. Liquid should cook down to a velvety consistency. (Add more chicken broth if needed.)

Serves 4
Approximately 116 calories per serving

Broccoli Rabe

1 bunch broccoli rabe, rinsed thoroughly
2 cloves garlic, minced
1/2 teaspoon Goya Adobo
1 tablespoon olive oil
1 cup of chicken broth

Rinse broccoli rabe in cold water and drain completely. Squeeze out excess liquid with hands. Trim stem bases off (about 2 inches). Chop broccoli rabe. Place oil and minced garlic in pot and sauté until garlic is light brown. Add chicken broth and stir in broccoli rabe, season with Goya and simmer for 4 to 7 minutes until tender.

Serves 3
Approximately 50 calories per serving

Honey is the only food that has an eternal shelf life. It will never go bad!

Roasted Roma Tomatoes

6 to 8 Roma tomatoes
  Reduced-fat mozzarella
  Parmesan cheese
  Seasoned bread crumbs
  Goya Adobo or sea salt and pepper to taste
1 tablespoon olive oil
1 tablespoon fresh basil

Slice Tomatoes about 1/4-inch-thick and toss in oil or use your sprayer. Place on non-stick baking sheet in a single layer. Sprinkle lightly with Goya and parmesan.

Bake at 375 for 20 minutes and remove from oven.

Place mozzarella on each one to cover and sprinkle lightly with a pinch of bread crumbs. Place back in the oven and bake until cheese melts, approximately 3 minutes.

Garnish with finely chopped basil.

Great Side Dish....

Serves 3 or 4
Approximately 150 calories per serving (for 3)
Approximately 115 calories per serving (for 4)

Steamed Green Veggies
They are a healthy, low-cal side that's always a plus in your diet choices.

Crisp Salad
Crisp Salad of your choice mixed in a lite dressing is another dish that is always a recommended healthy choice. We enjoy a fresh tomato and cucumber salad dressed in a lite balsamic vinaigrette.

SIMPLE CARB SIDES
Simple carb sides is where I am very aware of portion control. Simple carbs like white potatoes, white rice, pasta, and more are a concern. I may double up on my veggies, even my protein, but my sides of simple carbs are generally a single portion. You have seen where I have suggested to moderate "when necessary." This is what I have been talking about. It is necessary with the simple carbs for Steve and me to eat in moderation. However, I will double up on simple carbs (like for pasta, 4 ounces per serving instead of 2 ounces), for my dinner if it is part of the main entree. Other diets may require different foods to be consumed in moderation.

SNACKS

Pepperoni chips
Air popped popcorn
Pickles
Light n crisp Wasa crackers
Yogurt
Sugar snap peas (raw), a great sweet crunch
Medium apple with PB2
1 medium peach or Canned no sugar added peaches
2 medium kiwis
13 whole almonds
25 pistachios
2 slices toast (with low-cal no sugar added jelly and PB2) or
Cucumbers with PB2
In-the-shell Edamame
2 cups watermelon or 1/2 a cantaloupe
Any serving of most fruits
1/2 cup strawberries with whipped cream
1 cup of Swiss Miss hot chocolate
Sugar-free Jell-O Gelatin or Pudding
Crunchy Rice Rolls

And one of my favorites: 1/2 cup of Fiber One cereal with a serving of whipped cream in place of Almond milk. A few slices of peaches or a few berries added makes this little delight crazy good. Steve enjoys "Suzie's Corn, Quinoa and Sesame Thin Cakes" with Parkay Spray Butter in the evening. They are a great low-calorie crunchy treat. This is our list of foods in case we get hungry and we need something to hold us over until the next meal. It is not exhaustive. I am always searching and adding to our list. Because we are snackers, my guideline is to keep our snacks no more than 150 calories. The key here is portion control.

Pepperoni Chips

I want to tell you about them. They are as good as potato chips. So, in case your choice is a keto diet, or your snacks need to be protein, this is how you make them.

8 oz. pack of thinly sliced pepperoni

Pre-heat your oven to 350. Place your slices in a single layer on a non-stick baking sheet. Bake until crispy, about 10 to 15 minutes. Transfer your chips to paper towels. Sandwich them between two towels and press to absorb the fat if any.

Or you can place pepperoni single layered on a few paper towels on a paper plate. Cook for about 20 to 30 seconds in your microwave.

Remove them from the paper towels so they don't stick to the towels and let them cool and store in an air-tight container. (If there are any left.)

Enjoy!

Serves 2
Approximately 200 calories per serving

Your mind is a powerful thing. When you fill it with positive thoughts, your life will change.

DESSERT TIME
Ricotta Cups (Single Servings)

Version #1

1/2 cup of fat-free ricotta

2 teaspoon of Splenda

1 teaspoon of vanilla

Mix together and served chilled. Top with three large sliced strawberries and a dollop of whipped cream

Version #2

1/2 cup of fat-free ricotta

1/2 teaspoon of vanilla

1 teaspoon unsweetened cocoa powder

2 teaspoon Splenda

1 tablespoon slivered almonds

Mix and serve chilled. Top with whipped cream.

Version #3

1/2 cup fat-free ricotta

2 teaspoon Splenda

1/8 teaspoon cinnamon

1/8 teaspoon allspice

1/2 teaspoon vanilla

Mixed and serve chilled. Don't forget whipped cream!

Version #4

1/2 cup fat-free ricotta

1/2 teaspoon vanilla

1/4 teaspoon lemon juice

2 teaspoon Splenda

1 tablespoon shaved walnuts

Mix together and serve chilled.

Version #5 PB2 Time

1/2 cup fat-free ricotta

1/2 teaspoon vanilla

2 teaspoons Splenda

2 teaspoons PB2

Mix, serve chilled with whipped cream.

Have some fun. Try creating some of your own combinations.

Attention Keto dieters! Using whole milk ricotta makes for a great dessert for you.

Approximately 80 calories with fat-free and with nuts
Approximately 200 calories with part-skim and nuts
Approximately 245 calories with whole and nuts

Wintery Warm Peaches

14.5 ounce can no sugar added peaches

1/4 teaspoon cinnamon

1 tablespoon Splenda

1 tablespoon cornstarch

2 tablespoons raisins

  Whipped cream

1/4 cup water

Drain the peaches placing the liquid and water in a saucepan. Cut the peaches into bite-sized chunks and set them aside.

Add cinnamon, Splenda and cornstarch to the liquid in the saucepan. Bring to a boil, reduce heat and simmer while whisking continually until it thickens. Add peaches and raisins. Ready to serve... top with whipped cream.

Serves 2

Approximately 90 calories per serving

(This is great over 1/2 cup of no-sugar added vanilla ice cream. It would only add 80 calories per serving.)

Canned peaches were the first ever fruit to be consumed on the moon.

Fresh Strawberry Delight

1 pound of fresh strawberries, sliced
3 teaspoons Splenda
1/4 cup water

Place sliced strawberries, Splenda and water in a sealed plastic container. Shake vigorously for about 3 minutes.

Ready to serve ... top with whipped cream or pour 1/3 cup of strawberry delight over 1/2 cup of ice cream. Don't forget your whipped cream.

Serves 4
Approximately 60 calories per serving
With ice cream 140 per serving

A few tablespoons of this is yum over Michelly's Cheesecake (Page 133)!

1-2-3 Apple Pie

3 medium apples
2 teaspoons Splenda
1/4 teaspoon cinnamon
1 tablespoon Smart Balance Light
1/3 cup water
4 servings Ritz or club crackers

Peel and dice your apples. Place them in a sauce pan with Splenda, cinnamon, and water. Bring to a boil and reduce heat and simmer for 7 to 10 minutes until the apples are tender. Stir in Smart Balance. Be aware, that if you overcook, you will end up with a delicious apple sauce or apple jelly.

Break 1 serving size of club crackers in pieces in a small bowl and cover with your 1-2-3 apple pie mix ... you guessed it, eat. Top with a serving of whipped cream. And for an additional 60 calories, I top with a teaspoon of raisins and a teaspoon of shaved walnuts before adding the whipped cream.

Yummy served either warm or refrigerated!

Serves 4
Approximately 110 calories per serving

Make it a-la-mode with 1/4 cup sugar free ice cream at
Approximately 150 calories per serving

Fully loaded, it's only 210 calories per serving

NEED SOME CHOCOLATE?

SHOCKER ALERT!!! As a rule, we don't eat much chocolate. But this takes care of the chocolate attack when it occasionally strikes. That's only if there are no bite-sized Snickers in the galley.

60-Second Mug Cake (Single Serving)

3 tablespoons flour

3 tablespoons no-calorie sweetener

2 teaspoons cocoa powder

1/4 teaspoon baking powder

   Pinch salt

3 tablespoons milk

1 teaspoon vegetable oil

1 drop vanilla extract

Spray mug with a non-stick spray. In a separate bowl, combine your flour, sweetener, cocoa powder, baking powder and salt. Stir until there are no lumps remaining. Add milk, oil and vanilla and stir until smooth. Pour into cup and microwave for 60 seconds. You may need to adjust the time depending on your microwave. Note: don't overcook or it will be rubbery. Let it set for 2 to 3 minutes. Serve with powdered sugar, whipped topping, fruit, etc... It's your taste buds ... it's your choice.

You can of course, eat it from your mug. I drop mine on a plate, cut it horizontally, sprinkle a finely chopped walnut over both halves and top them with whipped topping... maybe lay it on a bed of sugar-free chocolate pudding.

SERIOUSLY... laying your halves in a shallow pool of sugar-free chocolate pudding would just change the calories a smidgen... yum.

Approximately 130 calories

Michelly's Cheesecake

16 ounces of fat-free cream cheese
1/3 cup fat-free ricotta
1/3 cup fat-free sour cream
4 tablespoons flour
2 egg whites
1 whole egg
1 teaspoon vanilla
3/4 cup Splenda
1/4 teaspoon salt
2 drops DoTerra essential lemon oil

Preheat oven to 350 and place a baking pan with 24 ounces of water on the lower oven rack. (This is to create a needed moisture in the oven when cooking a cheesecake.)

Put ingredients in a blender. Blend at high speed for approximately 3 minutes. Pour into a non-stick 8-inch springform pan. Cover with foil. Bake at 350 for an hour.

Let it cool in the oven for a couple of hours and then refrigerate overnight.

Serves 6
Approximately 130 calories per serving

We like to top ours with a few tablespoons of Crusty Crumbs (next page), a few tablespoons of Fresh Strawberry Delight and...a dollop of cool whip.

This recipe works great if you choose a keto plan. Just change all the "fat-free" to whole and use almond flour. If you choose to double the recipe, double the pan size and the cooking time.

Crusty Crumbs

2 cinnamon graham crackers
4 LaEstrella crackers (they have a crouton consistency)
3 tablespoons Splenda
1/4 teaspoon cinnamon
1/2 teaspoon cocoa powder
3 tablespoons slivered almonds

Combine ingredients in a blender and pulsate until you achieve a desired crumb consistency

I use this in place of crusts, sprinkling it on the top of cheesecakes, key lime pies, etc...

Approximately 315 calories per recipe

Chocolate was once used as currency!

Key Lime Pie

1/2 cup fat-free cottage cheese
1 key lime or lemon yogurt
1 lime Jell-O, sugar-free
4 tablespoons fat-free sour cream
8 tablespoons Cool Whip
8 ounces fat free cream cheese
1/4 teaspoon Stevia
4 tablespoon Splenda
8 drops DoTerra essential lemon oil
8 drops DoTerra essential lime oil

Combine in blender. Blend for approximately 3 minutes. Refrigerate overnight.

Top with crusty crumbs and whipping cream.

Serves 6
Approximately 155 calories per serving

BROWN SUGAR

1 cup Splenda
1 tablespoon molasses

Mix in blender. Makes 1/2 cup brown sugar. Keep refrigerated.

Approximately 60 calories per recipe

M&M's stand for Mars and Murry, the names of the two people who invented them.

OATMEAL RAISIN COOKIES

1-1/4 cup whole oats

1-1/4 cup oat flour (blender will flour whole oats)

1/2 cup brown sugar (page 136)

1/4 cup raisins

1/4 cup almond milk, 30-calorie

1/4 cup water

1 teaspoon vanilla

1 teaspoon cinnamon

1 teaspoon baking soda

1/2 teaspoon salt

1 teaspoon Stevia

2 tablespoon Smart Balance Light, melted

1 whole egg

Step 1 ... Soak raisins in water and almond milk and set aside.

Step 2 ... Combine whole oats, oat flour, cinnamon, baking soda, salt and stevia. Add brown sugar last and stir well.

Step 3 ... Separate the liquid from the raisins and place the liquid into a blender and the raisins into the dry mixture. Add to the raisin liquid in the blender; vanilla, melted butter, and egg and blend until well combined.

Combine Step 2 and 3 in large mixing bowl. Blend well with spatula. Let sit for just a few minutes (oats are absorbing and expanding).

Place spoonful drops on a baking sheet. Bake at 350 for 8 minutes.

Makes approximately 25 cookies
Approximately 48 calories per cookie

CARROT CAKE

2 egg whites
1 whole egg
1/4 cup almond milk, 30-calorie
1 cup no sugar added applesauce
1 teaspoon vanilla
2 teaspoon baking powder
1-1/2 teaspoons of cinnamon
1/4 teaspoon salt
1 teaspoon Stevia
1/2 cup brown sugar
2 cups oat flour (blender will flour whole oats)
1-1/2 cups carrots, about 3 to 4 medium carrots

Chop carrots in pulsing blender and set aside. In a mixing bowl combine oat flour, Stevia, salt, cinnamon and baking powder. Add brown sugar last and stir well.

Combine in a blender applesauce, vanilla, almond milk, egg whites and whole egg. Blend for not more than 10 seconds. (Do not overmix in the blender.)

Combine wet and dry ingredients. Stir well. Add carrots and stir. Fits well in an 8×8 baking pan sprayed with non-stick spray. Cook at 300 for 30 minutes.

Serves 6
Approximately 160 calories per serving
Top with cream cheese icing (Page 139)

CREAM CHEESE ICING
So easy.... So quick.... So yummy

8 ounces fat-free cream cheese
1/2 cup Splenda
2 tablespoon Smart Balance Light
2 teaspoon vanilla
3 tablespoon fat-free sour cream
1 teaspoon lemon juice or 1 drop DoTerra essential lemon oil

Mix in a blender until smooth. Refrigerate.

Makes approximately 18 servings
Approximately 20 calories per tablespoon

Apples are made up of 25% air, which is why they float!

Chapter 12 -- *Interviews*

Since we are not alone, I came up with these questions not to aid me with writing this book, but to show us all that we have more in common than one would think. I am including my questions and the interviews. After you read them, I believe you will see the commonalities that I expected to find.

I asked everyone who was interviewed the same basic questions, though some were asked additional questions according to their answers. Those interviewed were asked to be as truthful as they could be in order to help you with your personal search and so we could see that we are truly not alone.

I believe that you will find, as I did, that each had been required to make changes or adjustments, and that there is a commonality among us all. Our food battles, for the most part, are very similar. Whether a sweet tooth or bread lovers, it is safe to say that most us are carbohydrate addicts to some degree, trying to find our way.

As I spoke with others about their diets, I heard so many say that their food choices and habits were associated with past hurts and emotions. If this is you, it is a personal matter that should not be ignored.

FOR DIETERS:

- Prior to your found diet, what were you eating?
- When you decided to diet, did you look for a specific diet plan or was your diet self-created?
- What diet did you choose and why?
- How or where did you hear about the diet?
- What were the pros and cons?
- What were the results?

- What was your goal?
- Did you achieve it?
- If not, why do you think you didn't achieve your goal?
- Do you feel like you will be able to follow this diet indefinitely?
- Did you feel deprived of ANY foods that you enjoyed before this diet choice?
- Give an example of a breakfast, lunch and dinner. Do your lunches take extra time to prepare or are they just "grab and go" lunches?
- Realizing that family members have different likes, do the members of your household enjoy your dinner choice or do you prepare something different for them?
- Did you prepare the food yourself, or did you purchase pre-cooked meals and snacks through the mail?
- Has your health improved? Please explain.
- Would you recommend this weight loss choice to others?
- Are there any additional thoughts that you would like to add?

SURGICAL QUESTIONS:

- What type of surgical procedure did you elect?
- What were your given choices?
- What determined your choice?
- Did you encounter any complications?
- Were there immediate results? Positive or negative?
- Was there a diet plan that accompanied the procedure?
- Looking back, what do think were the pros and cons?
- Did you feel deprived of any foods that you enjoyed before the procedure?
- Give an example of breakfast, lunch and dinner.
- Do you eat differently than the rest of the family?
- What were the final results?
- Did you achieve your goal?

- Has your health improved? Explain.
- Would you recommend this procedure to others?
- Are there any additional thoughts that you would like to add?

I would suggest to you, the reader, that if you fit into either of these categories that you take a few minutes and answer the questions yourself. Be as honest as you can and then compare your answers to those that I interviewed. You may be surprised to find that you are not alone.

YOU'RE GOING TO BE AMAZED WITH THIS.
THIS IS KINDRA

Kindra is a fellow cruiser. In talking about the premise of this book, she stated that she intended to get started on a diet she had recently heard of. It was the Fast Metabolism Diet. I was intrigued, so I asked her if she would participate in the interviews. Her interview was so unique, I chose to give her answers verbatim.

Q... Prior to your found diet, what were you eating?
A... Anything I wanted.

Q... When you decided to diet, did you look for a specific diet plan or was it a self-created diet?
A... It was recommended by someone.

Q... What diet did you choose and why?
A... I chose the Fast Metabolism Diet, due to a possible 20-pound weight loss in 28 days. I liked the fact that it was based on stimulating your metabolism and viewed it as a jump start to a life change.

Q... How or where did you hear about this diet?
A... A lady started talking to me in the restroom of a tavern in the Florida Keys. She was one of the entertainers for the night. I had met her in passing once before.

Q... Were there any of your favorite foods on this plan?
A... I was attracted to the suggested recipes. There was a lot of Asian foods which I love.

Q... What were the pros and cons?
A... The pros were not having a lack of food due to eating 5 times a day. And the cons were having to eat 5 times per day, since I typically don't eat until mid-afternoon and a lot of times only at dinner time. And the type of food required multiple shopping trips during the week for fresh foods.

Q... What were the results?
A... I did not accomplish the diet. It was suggested that I start on a Monday. Shopping to get started just never took place

Q... What was your goal? Did you achieve it? If not, why do you think you didn't achieve your goal?
A... No, I did not achieve the desired 20-pound weight loss goal because instituting this diet with my family makeup was not conducive. My partner Bruce is very set in his food habit ways and this would have required two meals per sitting to accommodate his and my needs.

Q... Do you feel you would be able to continue to follow this diet indefinitely?
A... Not at this time, with failure under my belt and no success to go on

Q... Did you feel deprived of any foods that you enjoyed prior to this diet choice?
A... I don't think I would have felt deprived once I was seeing the results and getting past the processed sugars and carbs out of my daily regiment, since at one time in my life, I had eaten very clean and green and did not miss all the sugar that had once been there.

Q... Give an example of breakfast, lunch, and dinner.
A... I can't really speak about exact meals as I did not accomplish the diet, but it was about food combination,

protein and fruit one day and then a carbohydrate and protein another day. Rotating the food combinations was the premise of this diet to confuse and restart the metabolism in your body.

Q... Did you prepare the food yourself or did you purchase pre-cooked meals/snacks through the mail?
A... The diet would have been self-prepared.

Q... Would you recommend this weight-loss choice to others?
A... I can't really say however; I truly believe that it would have improved my health, and so I would have recommended it to others.

Q... Are there any additional thoughts you would like to add?
A... Yes. I have experienced the best results in my life from flushing my body with as much water as a gallon per day and cutting all refined sugars and carbs. Also, I have a deep belief in more small meals rather than starving your body, and although I am not adhering to it at this moment, I know and believe that this works.

This was the last question, but with the nature of her answer I needed to ask one more.

Q... Kindra, why, if you know and believe this works for you, what is your stopper from just doing it?
A... It's the endless gerbil wheel. It's instant gratification that makes me say to myself, "Forget this, I'm going to do what I want." Followed by, "I really, really, would enjoy this, this one time." Followed by endless self-sabotage in which I say to myself, "I tried to do good for a couple of days and I failed, so I might as well have what I want," which is the proverbial *endless gerbil wheel*.

What was so unique, you may ask? Kindra provided answers to a dieting questionnaire. A diet that she never started. Thank you so much, Kindra.

The purpose of the questionnaire is to share experiences. To help others make informed choices and to see that they're not alone.

I have heard a version of her answers over and over. How many times have you personally heard or said to yourself the "I'm going to" stories that never happen. She had a well-planned plan that never happened. And her reply to my last question I believe to be universal, not to mention brutally honest.

I believe everyone reading her answers will arrive at different conclusions. I would like to share mine.

We often hear of different diet plans that sounds so remarkable... and doable. There are many sources by which we gather information. Kindra was intrigued on a potty break. Come on, ladies, I know you've experienced that with one topic or another.

As I read the answer to the fifth question, this is where I feel she set herself up for failure though, of course, not realizing it. And I speak of failure with regard only to this particular plan.

She is now looking into a keto plan. This will blend more with both Kindra and Bruce. She mentioned that she has cut down on her carbohydrates already, but she's not quite sure how to make the change of no carbs. Kindra said that she had been on this food-battling gerbil wheel for the past year and she's ready to get off, and I believe she will.

The fast metabolism choice was not a failure. It was a stepping stone from going the wrong direction.

THIS ENTRY IS FROM PETER & KATHY

They are also fellow boaters. When I asked them to participate in the interviews, they were hesitant at first only because it had been years since their experience with the Atkins diet. Because keto plans are very popular today, coupled with my respect for the Dr. Atkins diet, I was quite anxious to hear their results from years ago.

Peter's response to, "What did you eat prior to starting the Atkins diet?" was (being a man of few words) the "see food" diet. What a great answer!!! I believe that his answer could be applicable to many prior to starting any plan.

Peter heard about Atkins from a friend who used it to prepare for a cruise. He chose this plan because it sounded like something he could follow. As he understood it, he could eat a lot of meat with no portion control, and that was appealing to him. He also remembered not being able to have caffeine or sugar, which was not so appealing. He shared that he grew up with desserts after dinner and had fond memories of his mom's homemade cookies every Tuesday.

I asked him about his breakfast, lunch and dinner menus. He mentioned meat and proteins for breakfast and dinner, but when it came to lunch his response was simply ... "no bread."

I know for a fact that there is more to the Atkins diet than protein, no bread and no caffeine. But in Peters memory, these are the things that stood out. Peter's wife Kathy, being the one who prepared meals, didn't really dive into the books' culinary suggestions. She said she just followed the basics. She did make mention of some delicious omelets that she prepared for breakfast with all the protein goodies.

As I chatted with Kathy, she said it was a pretty easy diet to prepare, in that you didn't have to figure out portions, but it soon got a bit boring...meat and veggies, meat and veggies. She said she was kind of glad when he stopped the plan. Although she herself was not on the Atkins diet, she missed making some of her favorite dishes such as casseroles made with pasta. She ate what she prepared for Peter, with a few carbohydrate additions to her plate. But her casseroles and dinners as such were on hold.

Although he did lose 20 pounds, they gradually came back.

In talking with him, he did mention that this was not something he could follow indefinitely, because there were too many restrictions.

Peter did want the readers to know, that for him, it was a quick way to see results and lose weight. For this reason, he would recommend it to others. Plus, it got him started on drinking diet pop instead of regular. Today he said he is trying to exercise and just eat smaller portions.

Thank you, guys....

MEET SUSANNE

She is one that found her way. I'm sure you're going to enjoy her interview as she shares her success in finding a plan she enjoys.

Sue is a member of Weight Watchers.

She was introduced to this program through television, and she heard good reports from her friend. One of the things that attracted her to Weight Watchers, was that she understood you could eat anything you wanted, that she just needed to learn portion control and decide if what she was choosing to eat was really worth it.

Prior to this found plan, Susanne mentioned that she had a nutritionist friend who schooled her in calories per day to help her drop weight. Although she did say it worked well, she didn't stick with it. During her interview, Susanne confessed her need for incentive and support which was found in the Weight Watchers Program.

Her initial goal was to lose 15 pounds. She reached her goal by changing her portions and changing out some food for less fat or less calories. And, she added, "This was without exercise".

Oh my goodness....changing portions? I asked if she was hungry as a result of eating SMALLER portions? Her answer was, "Not really. I just changed some of my food choices that would keep me full or that I could snack on if I was hungry."

I asked Susanne to give us examples of breakfast, lunch, and dinner.

Breakfast - corn flakes with almond milk and strawberries.
Lunch - deli turkey rolled up with cheese, sliced fruit or veggies dipped in hummus.
Dinner - chicken parmesan made with almond flour and baked in the oven with steamed veggies, potatoes, and a salad.

Susanne's husband's preferred foods are not as wide ranged as hers. Actually, Susanne said, "He's picky." She is able to prepare meals that they both enjoy. Sue follows a gluten free diet and stays away, for the most part, from processed foods. She has been able to incorporate her personal food choices into this program.

When I asked if her health has improved, her response was, "When I stick with it, I feel better and I have more energy." I think that's a great report. I then asked, "Why don't you stick with it?"

As Susanne explained, her chosen plan was so easy and comfortable for her, that she would slack off from attending meetings and lose her way. Her diet became so automatic. This is such a good thing but there went her needed "incentive and support," and so her accountability was gone as well.

She stated that she went back to eating too fast, stopped paying attention to portion control and well.... then there was THAT ice cream....one frozen delight, and then another, and soon she found herself on the ice cream path to regaining those lost pounds.

(I've got to say, "I'm also all about those frozen delights. I'm right alongside of you, girlfriend.")

But because Susanne found a plan that fit her so well, getting back on track has not been an issue. She's been with Weight Watchers since 2010. She doesn't feel deprived of any foods, and she would recommend it to others.

At the completion of her interview, I asked her to share the cons with us. She said there were none. So I asked again, saying, "Nothing I know is perfect; isn't there one thing that comes to mind?"

Susanne said, "No, nothing."

And lastly, I asked, "Do you feel you can follow this plan indefinitely?" "Yes," she said, "because, I do take breaks and *fall off the wagon* at times. But I always know I can go back and fix it."

Awesome testimonial, Sue.

TIME TO VISIT NEW YORK KAREN

Karen shared about her Atkins experience. She was on this plan for six weeks, a year ago, at the time of her interview

Prior to starting her Atkins diet, Karen said she ate a lot of bread, too much bread, and just too many carbs in general. She mentioned that she looked into the South Beach Diet, but it didn't seem feasible for her to stick to it because she's basically a carnivore. She loves meat, and so the Atkins diet seemed to fit her better.

She heard about both of these particular diets through talking with friends.

When I asked Karen to share the pros and cons, she addressed the cons first. What came to mind was the discomfort that she felt adjusting to the new diet. It was an uncomfortable feeling in her stomach, somewhat like a diarrhea queasiness. She attributed this to her body needing time to adjust to the diet change. She felt this was also due to a type of cleansing this change provided which took a few days. She added that she missed her breads, wine, and chocolate. Remember, Karen is from New York. She's a bagel lover, too. She is a carnivore who loves bagels.

And so, what are the pros? It's very simple, really. As we chatted, Karen talked about the different meals that she was able to enjoy eating and her willingness to give up the breads, her sweets and her wine for a period, until she could slowly incorporate them back into her diet.

The results were that she had more energy and she achieved her goal of losing 15 pounds. But she did continue with, "It was great at first, but 6 weeks into it, I kind of got tired of what I was required to eat."

Her examples of meals were:
Breakfast – "Ham 'n cheese omelets, with bacon or sausage ... all sorts of lovely things."
Lunch - burgers with bacon and cheese no bread. A grab-and-go lunch would be rollups. (A simple roll-up is a slice of cheese rolled up in a lunch meat of choice.)
Dinner - shrimp, fish or meat.

She made mention of being sad that she was not allowed to have ketchup on some of her omelets.... but she added, "You need to compromise so I throw a little black pepper on top."

Karen said, "You get to eat half of really what you want to eat. Like lunch, with burgers and bacon and cheese... but no bread. But it's okay, because the burgers were delicious."

"I followed it very strictly. I used ketone strips to check myself. They were a great reinforcement for me. Using the ketone strips helps keep you on track even if the scale hasn't changed yet."

When asked if she would recommend this plan to others, her reply was, "Definitely, it works if you follow it, but you have to follow it." Her thoughts were.... it's about how much weight you want to lose, how long can you stay on the diet and that's different for everybody.

Today, she has limited breads in her galley/kitchen and she eats a modified version of her Atkins experience. Her diet is of her own modifications and she feels she is more protein and less carb minded these days...that's not to say that she doesn't enjoy a New York bagel now and then.

TIRED OF THE WAY YOU SEE YOURSELF? ROSALIE WAS TOO

Rosalie is a high school bestie of mine.

Life doesn't always go as planned for so many. As we talked through the interview pertaining to diets, I was aware it was difficult for her to separate her eating habits from her emotions... have you come across that issue in ***Time to Stop the Battle (Eating with Freedom)*** yet. It's throughout the pages.

My friend said she was very unhappy in her personal life and with herself. Due to Rosalie's unhappiness, she found herself eating whatever she wanted. The excess weight was gathering around her stomach. And now she was also very unhappy with the way she looked. She got to a point where enough was enough. She needed to do something. So, she started doing her own thing, a self-created plan.

I asked her how many diet plans she thought that she had been on in the past 25 years. She said, "Michele, if I have to guess, oh, at least 50," she went on to say, "I have tried everything from shakes, to pills, to starvation, to Weight Watchers, and Nutrisystem. I've tried herbs, I've tried teas, I've tried everything."

Q... What served you best?
A... Exercise routines and walking started me in the right direction. Being an emotional eater, it provided peace of mind, a calm feeling and a pride that I was finally moving in the right direction. I started going to the gym, and at home I would dance to music and do sit-ups. I did all sorts of things.

Heart disease and diabetes were in her family tree. Many of her choices derived from these issues. She searched for a healthier way, so as not to fall into her family's medical pattern. She found no negative issues with her choices. Through this self-created plan, she met her goal. She felt better, looked better, and had more energy.

Q... You feel better. Would you say your health has improved?
A... The doctor said my blood work is impeccable and I never have to worry about being a diabetic.

Q... How did your eating change?
A... I started eating healthier. I stayed away from fast foods totally. I ate more chicken, fish, vegetable pasta and no sodas, just water. In the morning I drink lemon water which kicks up my metabolism. I found myself to be less hungry. I enjoy a lot of vegetables and salads. I don't eat junk anymore. It's not that I never eat it, I don't deprive myself. If I'm out and I want dessert, I have it. I don't have a piece of cake or pie or a bag of chips every night. It's just not the first thing I grab anymore. You can't tell yourself you'll never have

those foods you stay away from, you'll never do it. I would have never been able to stick to it with that mindset.

Rosalie shared that she went from 196 to 135 pounds. She would like to see herself at 125 pounds. She has decided to try the Keto Diet to drop that last 10 pounds. Rosalie continues to do today what she did from the start of her plan. She's an early riser who walks approximately 5 miles a day prior to the start of her workday.

When I asked Roe if she had any additional thoughts, she gave us this, "It takes time. You can't give up. You may have to give up some things, but not all at once just a little at a time. Feel positive about yourself. You can do this. Don't tell yourself, 'I've tried a million diets. Nothing's going to work.' It will work."

NOT THE NORM
DARLENE STAYED ON TOP OF HER BATTLE

We all have so much in common, yet I am amazed at our differences.

This is my sister, Darlene. I believe when you read her interview, it may appear that her battle is minimal. Never having been on a specific diet plan, Darlene, like our mother, has held her weight between approximately 135 and 155 pounds.

She said that when she reached her heaviest at 155 pounds, it frightened her because she knew she could easily continue to keep going upward in that direction. "I didn't realize how much weight came on me until I really looked at myself, and I didn't like it."

Some of her favorite foods are fettuccine, pizza and crusty breads. She said, "But I don't eat them very often. I could live on crusty bread and butter. But I don't."

Q... Why don't you eat your favorite foods that often?
A... I don't want to eat carbs that often. But I do enjoy a large variety of food; the list is long. Homemade soups are on the list, vegetable and chicken soups in particular. I have come across a few velvety soups that I'm really enjoying. This is one of them."

5 medium carrots cut into 2-inch pieces
6 cups of chicken broth
2 large potatoes, cubed
1 medium onion
Add together in a pot and bring to boil. Simmer until tender. Puree in a blender. Add 2 to 3 teaspoons of brown sugar, Goya seasoning or salt, and pepper to taste and one can of cream of mushroom soup. Blend together once more.

(I tried this, and like Darlene, I enjoyed it. I recommend trying it on a cold winter day. It will warm your inner *shiver to the bone* away.)

Dar continued, "I really don't eat anything in particular that often. I have no regimen, except for my breakfast. I blend an energy drink for breakfast. Lunch is soup, sandwich or salad. And for dinner, I go by the seat of my pants. Whatever I'm in the mood for."

Q... To what do you attribute the long list of foods that you enjoy today?
A... Definitely my childhood. We grew up with a variety of food that were mixed together. Also, we were taught to try everything whether we liked it or not, whether we wanted to or not.

Q... What did you do when you got uncomfortable with your weight gain?
A... I stopped eating at McDonald's (I really enjoy burgers), and drinking sodas I just started eating differently. I watched my carbs to some degree. I could eat a lot of food, but I learned to taste what I was eating which helped downsize

the amount of food I consumed. I'll sometimes take the cheese off of pizza... things like that to cut calories. I always cook for myself, so I can keep things in balance. I drink a lot of carbonated water. That's filling. And I got back on track with exercise. Exercise has always been a part of my life, and I believe it is a key element in remaining healthy.

Q... So, did you feel deprived of foods you enjoy?
A... Not so much deprived, but I do discipline myself. I am a night time snacker like my sister. I like shoveling food in my mouth late at night.... but I don't. If I snack, I make sure its light.

Q... Was it a struggle?
A... Not so much... because I had my eye on the benefits. I knew what they were.

Q... What motivated you to stop that upward climb on the scale?
A... A mind-set came about. Shame on me if I'm not willing to do what's necessary to stay healthy. I believe it's a responsibility that we have. I believe that what we have been given, we need to take care of. I look at it from that perspective. Darlene finished by saying, "Energy is a key for me. If I don't have energy, I don't have me. I may never reach where I would like to be, but I will continue to work towards a goal of staying somewhat fit".

SOPHIA KEPT IT REAL

I began by asking Sophia, just as I had asked others, "How many diets do you think you've been on in the last 25 years or so?"

That was a good start. She said, "I don't know, maybe 3. Back in the day, I was on Weight Watchers for 12 years and kept the weight off. I feel it's one of the best programs available. It's just not working for me in this stage of my life. I quit smoking cigarettes and blame that for my eating habits because I substituted food for cigarettes. I gained it all back. That went on for a long time."

"I believe I ate healthy, but I just ate too much, and sometimes I would binge. I am a volume eater as well as an emotional eater. I actually doubled the weight I had lost."

"I didn't go crazy on the junk food because of my Weight Watchers background. I was doing okay during the week, but the weekends I would go all out."

"About 3 years ago I paid for a trainer, and they gave me a food plan. I really needed to invest in myself."

"The food plan was a lot of chicken, fish, baked potatoes, and I had a cheat day one day a week."

"It worked. I lost a lot of inches between working out and eating. Again, I was losing inches working with the trainer, but it took eight months to lose 12 pounds and I was going two to three times a week, and the trainer was a bit pricey for me."

"One morning I woke up, and my arms and legs were very sore. I couldn't raise my arms in church for 3 months in praise to my Lord."

"I talked to my trainer about my physical soreness. I told her, 'I can't lift my arms, I'm in pain.' Stretching and working it out helped, but when my body relaxed at home, it was still very painful to stand from a sitting position off the sofa."

"This discomfort was affecting my work. I can't work with that level of discomfort. Although I did stay on their food program for a while, it needed to come to an end."

"This was my LA/Fitness experience. I was the heaviest I had ever been when I started at LA/Fitness. It was a little disappointing to say the least because I felt I was working so hard at it."

Sophia very much appreciated her trainer. She felt her trainer was very attentive to her issues. It just wasn't working for her.

"My pastor invited me to a meeting to introduce me to Optavia. He looked great, and I was aware that quite a few other church members had also lost significant amounts of weight. I made a decision. I was going to try this. I'm going to give it a month. After all, this wasn't a commercial I saw on TV. I was actually seeing others at my church that I knew, losing significant amounts of weight."

Sophia's results... she has been on Optavia about a year.

Q... What were the pros on this program?
A... IT WORKS. The weight started coming off immediately. It's easy, it's quick, and I know what I have to eat. It's a grab & go and super convenient for me. In the beginning there are encouraging videos. They are very short. I really like them. There are a lot of helpful resources and you have a life coach. If you have any questions, there is always someone available to answer. I feel good and I have more energy, simply because of not being so heavy. Getting on the scale is the best. I lost 50 pounds in 7 months. Another pro, and this is a big one, I'M OUT OF THE PLUS SIZES.

Q... What are the cons?
A... You do get hungry, especially if you're a volume eater like me. It's hard in the beginning to get used to drinking a lot of water. But after a while, you're thirsty all the time. The water intake gets easier. And I don't like some of the packaged food. To me, the food is very bland. I'm Latin; bland food really doesn't work well for me. (You can add your own seasoning sometimes... but still, the food ends up quite bland.) I like to taste something. I also found that parties are not very easy. There's always a tasty variety of foods at parties.

Q... Do you think you can be on this diet indefinitely?
A... I really don't know. I have to do something. I don't want to gain my weight back ever again.

Q... Do you feel deprived of any of the foods that you enjoy?
A... Ahhh....YEAH...LOL.... Really? If somebody says no, they are just lying. Give me a break. Are you kidding? I didn't eat bread or rice for months. Yeah, of course you're going to feel deprived of things. But what are your priorities? It's a decision. It's a choice.

Q... Would you recommend this program to others?
A... Yes, yes, and again yes. I have already recommended this to a couple of people and they have had good results. But I tell them that the whole thing is you have to be determined to do it. It works if you do the plan the way you're supposed to. Right now, I'm on a sabbatical. I am half on and half off.

Q... What does that look like, Sophia?
A... At dinner, instead of veggies, I may have bread-and-butter. I love my bread. Maybe mashed potatoes, rice or piece of cake. And if I go out on the weekends, I'll have what is offered. It seems like things are always popping up around my food plans. It can make it difficult to stay on it. But I am maintaining. I am planning to go back on 100%. I want to get off the rest of this weight. They do have a maintenance program, but I am not familiar with it as of yet.

Sophia finished with, "I am not where I want to be, but at least I know that there's something that works for me. At this stage of my life, that makes a big difference."

TALKING TO PATTY WAS AN UNEXPECTED HOOT

I called my good friend Patty, reminding her about our planned interview. She was very reluctant to do the interview to say the least.

We have worked together, multi-leveled together, chubbed out together, and dieted together.

After we said our hellos, she said, "You don't want to interview me, I'm the worst person to ask questions about a diet right now. I look like a _ _ _ _ _ _ _. I have gained so much weight." My response was, "On the contrary. You're just like so many others. You're exactly who I want to interview. People need to know they are not alone."

With frustration she added, "How am I supposed to do an interview? I can't even remember that stupid 17-day diet I said we would talk about. It's been so long ago."

"I really want to start something new anyway. I've got to do something. I'm so fed up. I'm not even eating junk food. And I find myself gaining weight anyway. I'm presently working a lot of hours, and by the time I get home it's too late to eat or prepare a proper meal. It's a battle."

So we chatted awhile. We talked about different diets. We talked about the pitfalls of the "yo-yo", lose and gain. That one way or another we all have similar reasons for not doing or following what we know works. And for some of us, not being our used to be "young selves" makes it even a little harder to drop the weight.

She attributes some of her recent weight gain to the removal of her gallbladder. Today, Patty's thoughts on fast losing diets are that most often they result in a fast regaining of those lost pounds.

So many share Patty's frustrations. I was successful in convincing her that people need to hear from her.

So, this is Patty's interview.

About 3 years ago she heard about the 17-Day Diet on one of the talk shows. Patty and her husband completed and actually went a little beyond the 17 days.

I asked Patty what intrigued her that she heard that day...... and the laughter begins .... she answered, "I liked the name of it. Seventeen days sounded good to me."

Q... What were the results?
A... We lost a little weight. I appreciated doing it with my husband. It was fun having someone to share it with.

Q... Did you have a goal?
A... I wanted to feel better. I didn't want to feel so bloated. I wanted to fit in my clothes. And it did work, but it seemed to work better for my husband. I think men lose easier and quicker than women.

Patty remembers that it was strict in the beginning, and there were levels. It was very limited, basically veggies, protein, and a lot of water. After the first week you could introduce foods that you couldn't have initially. She said, "I prepared our meals myself. I'm not a fan of pre-packaged foods. I'd rather cook it myself, this way I know what I'm eating."

We giggled ourselves silly on this next one!

Q... Did you feel deprived of any foods?
A... Yeah.... of course.... I wouldn't need to be on a diet if I could eat everything I wanted.... THAT WAS A STUPID QUESTION, MICHELE! LOL!

Okay, let me reword the question.
Q... Was there anything in particular that you missed during this plan?

A... I'm trying to think back to everything you CAN'T have: you can't have bread, you can't have ice cream, and you can't have doughnuts, etc. I guess not being able to have bread was the worst thing. I love my bread.

I asked her if she would recommend this plan to others. She said, "I think I would, but it all depends how disciplined you are. Once you achieve your goal, you need to stick with it. I guess that's with any diet. But I personally got to a point after losing the weight, thinking, well I can have this now, I haven't had it in a while. I didn't gain so I can have this too. Again, nothing happened, so, I can have that also. And slowly but surely, I started to put the weight back on, and here I am again trying to do something else. Temptation, stress, and sometimes normal issues in life are what can cause the best diet to fall short.

In the past, Patty enjoyed and had success with the South Beach diet and Somersizing with Suzanne Somers. She's contemplating Somersizing again.

As our talk continued, I asked her if she had any final thoughts to share. After some thought, Patty said, "Yes...... basically, you have to do what you feel is the right diet for you. You're going to hear about many other diets that people have gone through. You have to do what feels comfortable within your own skin. Everybody's weight issues are different, everybody's health issues are different, and everybody thinks differently. Do what feels right."

KRISTIES SEARCH

Over the years, there have been many diets come across her path. She has tried Medifast, Atkins, Nutrisystem, the Bariatric Diet, she touched on Weight Watchers and the blood type diet to control her weight and wellness. She recently started Juice Plus. Kristie is very health conscious of herself and family.

In this interview she and I will be talking about the blood type diet by Doctor Peter D'Adamo.

I started this interview with the first question I've asked everybody. That question is, "What were you eating prior to this found diet?" Kristie said, "Mostly anything I felt like eating: carbs, sweets, you name it, but always in moderation. I would only eat small portions and I would eat five times a day."

Q... Why small portions? 5 times a day?
A... Well, from what I read about suppressing hunger, consuming smaller portions 5 times a day curbs your appetite from getting out of control. I knew medically from personal research that is the healthier way to go.

But she just didn't feel healthy or energetic. She also was a coffee drinker two to three times a day.

Kristie was interested in knowing what specific foods were best for her. At this point she was not interested in what fad diet was popular at the time. She shared that Doctor D'Adamo believes that each blood type's unique antigen marker reacts to certain foods. If the wrong foods are consumed, it can lead to a host of health problems. Doctor D'Adamo also believes that stomach acid levels and digestive enzymes are associated with blood type. By eating foods compatible to your blood type, you may digest and absorb nutrients more efficiently. This results in optimal health and weight loss. Each blood type has its own unique diet and exercise prescription including recommended foods and foods/food groups to avoid.

She stumbled upon this information on a webinar series online by Dr. D'Adamo.

When asked to share the pros and cons, Kristie started with the cons as most people do. Kristie felt it was very complicated and time consuming to learn. The diet was very restrictive as far as what foods were actually consumable according to her blood type, which is o-negative. She said that according to her blood type, her diet should have basically been gluten free and dairy free. She also found it expensive to buy all organic foods and the recommended meats that are lean, grass-fed, organic, and range free which, besides being expensive, are difficult to find. Oh.... and she missed cheese the most.

With the above being said, Kristie found the results to be very positive. She stopped drinking coffee because of this diet and said she feels much better since she eliminated coffee from her system. She shared that the foods that you do consume are very healthy, whole, and unprocessed, and it makes you feel amazing. Her mind was its sharpest and her head felt very focused and clear. She had great energy, she slept well, and felt great. As she put it, "I had plenty of exercise energy, so working out wasn't such a strain." She lost 10 pounds over the 6 weeks that she followed the diet.

Q... Why did you follow this diet only 6 weeks?
A... It is extremely difficult to follow. It was very expensive, and I didn't really like dropping the foods that I had to eliminate. It was very specific and limited on certain foods in which I had to both choose from and eliminate.

Q... Did you achieve your goal?
A... I did, but after the diet, I gained back 20 pounds, so now I'm heavier than before I started.

Q... To what do you attribute your weight gain after the 6 weeks?
A... Stress, emotional eating and lack of 'follow-through' and discipline.

Today she still tends to gravitate toward the foods that were on the beneficial list and finds she feels better when eating them. She believes the diet is correct in its assessment, it's just that in today's society it's difficult to follow.

Here are some examples of her foods through the day. For breakfast she would have a couple of scrambled eggs, sometimes Ezekiel toast and some fruit. She would have a small snack in the morning of either pumpkin seeds or veggies. Lunch was something gluten-free and dairy-free. Kristie often works on the road, so she said she would generally find something to take with her or buy lunch in her travels. She said that usually one of the franchises like Panera Bread or Wawa would have what she needed. Dinner generally came from a cookbook that she bought that accompanies the diet.

Her family enjoyed the recipes from the cookbook. Kristie would just add a grain or two for her family even though she wouldn't eat it. When asked if she would recommend this plan, she said, "Absolutely. Yes, it was not the easiest for me... but that was me. The science behind it makes sense. I believe in the philosophy of it and I feel it would be beneficial for people to look into it."

Kristie told me that she has always battled with a form of Irritable Bowel Syndrome. I'm so glad she mentioned this in a follow-up conversation we had a few weeks later. Although she felt her best with the blood type diet, it wasn't feasible for her, and it didn't take care of all her needs.

Since the initial interview, she has come across Juice Plus, which has helped her with her immensely with her IBS. (You can read about Juice Plus in Tina's blog at the end of this chapter.)

At present, Kristie is keeping a close watch on her carb intake. She is staying away from bready gluttonous foods because they tend to slow her down mentally.

"I'm eating 5 small meals through the day. That's the basics, I'm taking my Juice Plus supplements and I'm drinking lots of water."

> For me, at the age of 14, I was diagnosed with hypoglycemia, and my doctor recommended that I eat six small meals through the day. I'm very grateful that I am no longer afflicted with hypoglycemia. Through the years, I have also heard this advice given to others to aide in different health issues. It is a concept worth looking into for herself.

INTERVIEWING TONA

Let's start with Tona's background story.

As you will discover, Tona didn't stop with her search. I am convinced that many will feel they have walked in her shoes.

Tona started our discussion with a giggle, saying, "It was easy to lose weight when I was single." "In the past," she said, "I tried being a vegetarian, fad diets, the soup diet, Weight Watchers, Slim-Fast, this diet, that diet, you name it."

She shared that back in the day when she was first saved, there was a huge movement in the Christian faith. It was to eat only the foods mentioned in the bible. She took it one step further and became a vegetarian.

She lost an enormous amount of weight, becoming anorexia thin. She developed a mercury deficiency. Her doctor said that being a vegetarian was not a good choice for her, so she went back to eating regular food. I had to ask:

Q... What is regular food?
A... Regular food is what you eat when you're not on a specific diet plan. And much to her children's happiness, they said, we don't have to eat nuts and berries anymore.

And so, we continued. She then started Weight Watchers. Tona met her goal and became a leader. And again, she was successful in losing her weight, but felt that they set her goal way too low for her body frame. She said, "People would say to me, 'Tona, you look like Nancy Reagan.' Your head is too big for your body."

She maintained her weight for a few years. Adding exercise to her plan created changes in her body frame, and she gained enough weight to put her on the wrong side of her goal weight. Although it is not like this anymore, back in the day, a leader was required to maintain their goal weight.

Staying within those rigid requirements was a real struggle for her, so she gave up and Weight Watchers went by the wayside. And, of course, the weight returned.

Atkins was her next endeavor. She developed some health issues and after needed surgery, her doctor advised her to discontinue with that plan. Tona kept going. She gave Weight Watchers another try. But the new plan was not for her.

She tried SlimFast for six months. Let's dive into her experience with this plan.

Prior to starting SlimFast, Tona was consuming "regular food" with her family. (Remember, regular food is eating foods that are not in a diet plan.) **Too funny, Tona....**

She found it simple and easy. When she was younger on this plan, she craved chocolate. SlimFast had a chocolate shake that took care of that. She said the shake was one of the reasons she chose the program.

So, for breakfast and lunch she would drink a shake and then for dinner she would have a portion-sized meal. She found it very simple for a working mom.

I asked her if it was satisfying, and she immediately said, "Absolutely...not. It wasn't enough of anything. I was hungry an hour and a half later. And when dinner time came around and it was portion sized.... ugh. My boys would always tease me and say, 'Great mom, more for us.'"

She continued to share, that at the dinner table, there were foods on the table, in front of her, such as potatoes, deserts, and more, which were not going on her plate. She would dish out, for her family, food that was not in her plan. Her dinner was generally a meat and some green veggies. She shared that her finances didn't enable her to purchase special foods and veggies to produce variety. It was really hard. She lost about 15 pounds. It wasn't much, and she didn't feel any better. And she added, "Disposition wise, I was probably grumpy. I think my kids would attest to that." It wasn't satisfying, and she found it boring. Tona shared that food and flavor is important. If you're not enjoying the food you eat, why eat it? And, it was always in the back of her mind that drinking your meals was not really a healthy way to live.

Well, this is some of Tona's food battle journey. I know I've been there.

I asked her if she had any final thoughts to share. "Unfortunately, I feel a lot of these diets have a gimmick of some sort. I don't think they started out that way. But they aren't a good path for everyone. There are people from all different cultures. How is it possible for it to work for everybody? Every diet is not necessarily the best thing for everyone. Most diets recommend eating breakfast. That just doesn't work for me."

Today, Tona plans to continue her search. Her plan is to find her way according to who she is. She felt that ***Time to Stop the Battle" (Eating with Freedom)*** may be the key for her.

A MARRIED COUPLE'S SHARED EXPERIENCE CINDY AND AL

Being personal acquaintances for many years, I would say that Alfred is my Italian friend. We're talking a heavy pasta background among many other Italian delicacies like cannoli and the like. Need I say more? I would say (and have said) that my friend Cindy was the poster child for "Sara Lee" pastries.

I interviewed them separately. Let's look at what they found works for them.

Q... So, what did you guys eat prior to this found diet?
A... Cindy said, "Pasta, bread, and desserts, fruits and veggies.... not a lot of processed food."
A... Al said, "Everything and anything."

They heard about this diet from Pastor Anthony. You can review his blog at the end of this chapter. It was from a book suggested by Pastor Anthony's son called *Fat for Fuel* written by Dr. Joseph Mercola.

There were 4 couples who were planning to try this together. Al shared that he thought it is better when there's a joint or team effort supporting one another. Only two of the couples stayed with it. And as you read on, you'll see that they continued with great success. The other two couples were not convinced for different reasons. They tried the diet and found it wasn't for them.

Q... Why did you choose this diet?
A... Cindy - I like eating avocados and the idea of eating good fats. And I found it easy to follow.
A... Al - I understood the diet after a fast I was on. During this fast when I stopped consuming carbs, I noticed the feeling of being hungry minimized considerably.

Q... What were the pros and cons? Let's start with some of the struggles.
A... Cindy - Not being able to have carbs like pasta and bread. That was hard to give up, and of course sugar in general is hard to give up.
A... Al - now Al had a little bit more to say about this. He shared that you're limited as to what you can eat. There's no snacks.... No chips, no pretzels, besides maybe a handful of nuts and just certain nuts. You can't have a nice apple pie or a slice of lemon meringue. Now Cindy has been making a no-carb bread and even Stromboli. There are fat bombs made with dark chocolate if you need something for a sweet tooth. But as far as snacks, you can have some pepperoni and cheese, or you can chew on some olives or nuts.

Q... At the start, what were the pros and pluses you noticed?
A... Cindy - More energy, immediate weight loss, and the feeling of hunger greatly diminished.
A... Al - LOL... My friend Al said, "I got to eat all the meat and fat I wanted that Cindy was telling me over the years I could not or should not have."

Got to love that Alfred.

Al lost 25 pounds and Cindy was down 30 pounds in the first 5 months. Cindy was only shy 3 pounds of her goal. When I asked Alfred if he had a goal, his answer was, "No, I just wanted to lose weight because I couldn't bend over to tie my shoes."

Got to love that Alfred.

Q... Do you think you can continue this diet indefinitely? Although I interviewed them separately their answers, we're exactly the same for this question They said....
A... "Absolutely, it's been almost a year; it's a lifestyle now."

Q... Do you feel deprived of any foods that you enjoyed prior to this diet?
A... Cindy - Once in a while. I really don't deprive myself. If I want a bowl of pasta, I'll have some but maybe 1/4 of what I used to have. I really only did that once. I'm satisfied that way. I'm not going to do without if I really want something.
A... Al - Well you can't have pasta and bread. You can't have French toast or pancakes. I have watched my mother on insulin with her diabetic battle. My niece at 36 is a pre-diabetic. I don't ever want to get to that point. So, if I have to make a few changes in my life, I'd rather do that than have to take pills and pinch needles for the rest of my life. I don't want to eat food that's not healthy for me now which would cause me later on in life to have regrets.

For breakfast, they both talked about pork roll, egg, and cheese or bacon, egg, and cheese which, Cindy added, 'Is cooked in butter and coconut oil.' I'm thinking ...What about sausage? I'm a sausage girl myself.

Getting back to Cindy and Al. They also both talked about a drink for breakfast called a bullet. I understand that it's a tablespoon of butter, a tablespoon of coconut oil, a tablespoon of heavy cream, a raw egg with Xylitol for a sweetener. This is whipped in a cup of coffee. Cindy said it is loaded with all good fats. Al said it tastes good like a milkshake. This drink is a breakfast in itself and they said it will hold them over till 1 or 2 in the afternoon.

I must confess, I pushed a bit with my old friend "Sara Lee". I asked her, "Cindy, don't you miss pancakes or French toast?" But Sara Lee wasn't there. Cindy answered, "No I haven't missed any of that. My big miss is breads. But I make my own bread, actually two types and they're very good."

And so, I moved on to lunch.

Cindy - I like a big salad. You can have any kind of block cheese and maybe some chicken breast. You can have a loaded salad. My personal choice for dressing is either blue cheese or olive oil with lemon.
Al - I like a sub in the tub. Of course, that's just a sub with no bread. Or I'll have a cold cut mix, maybe roast beef and cheese. With that I'll hit the olive bar if one is available.

For dinner, Al shared that Cindy makes everything, just normal dinners. He continued by saying, "The other night Cindy made a casserole with chicken breast, cream cheese, mozzarella and spinach. It was delicious. Cindy tries to serve 3 quarters of the plate with green veggies and just 4 ounces of a protein. Of course, you can have more of both." They have grass-fed meats delivered to their home.

Q... Has your health improved?
A... Cindy - My blood lab levels are normal to good. My energy level is up. I have an overall wellness. I have no complaints.
A... Al - Cindy almost fell off the chair. My blood levels were 10 times better than hers. I feel good and I have more energy. When my blood work came back, she couldn't believe it. My blood levels came out perfect.

Got to love that Alfred.

They would both highly recommend this to others. Cindy added, "Especially to diabetics."

I asked them if they would like to share any additional thoughts. Cindy mentioned that the book by Dr. Joseph Mercola, *Fat for Fuel*, teaches you how good fats affect your cells. She added, "If you choose this way of eating, it must become a lifestyle. There are recipes to help you make the transition. Recipes that show you how to make your own pasta and breads."

Al said, "Push away all that sugar and keep mindful of your carbs. That's all you have to do. And most importantly," Al added, "God gave you a body and asked you to take care of it. If you're not doing that, you're not doing it justice."

MEDICAL PROCEDURE INTERVIEWS

The medical information given here may not necessarily be exhaustive or medically accurate, given the fact that the interviewees are not part of the medical field, nor am I, but how the interviewees perceived or understood the information given them. However, their experience is accurate. And, although the number of interviews is few, they all had some similar issues but no regrets about having had the procedure done.

LUPE HAS BEEN THERE AND BACK

At the time of Lupe's interview, four years have gone by since her surgery. She chose a gastric sleeve. Because of an abnormality in her heart, and thyroidism at the time of her Body Mass Index (BMI), she was told that she was less than six months away from becoming a full-blown diabetic.

She tried a weight-loss medication. The medication was Qsymia. It was a medication for migraines and depression. One of its side effects was an appetite suppressant. It was rebranded the "Obesity Pill" and was extremely expensive.

She did this for about a year. There were more side effects in store for Lupe. It started with a numbness. Lupe had trouble sleeping and had tingling in her hands and feet. In addition, her entire left side was going numb. Lupe said, "I was not losing any weight; it was time to stop."

"Dieting didn't work for me because of my lifestyle, my level of stress, and a few health issues. And the why I was overweight I would later learn of."

Lupe started searching out bariatric surgery and learned that there were three types of surgeries under the umbrella of bariatric surgery.

There were multiple reasons mentioned for Lupe's belief that the gastric sleeve was the best choice for her out of the three. One of the important factors was the fact that she is a cancer survivor and her family has a bad history of stomach illnesses. These were issues that needed to be considered when choosing.

One of the things that Lupe found appealing about the gastric sleeve was that it completely removed 3/4 of the stomach, leaving her with a normal body and a smaller stomach.

Her stay in the hospital was less than 24 hours. She said there was absolutely no pain, and she was home by the 20th hour. Surgery was performed through three minor little holes. It's always a point of interest to know that there were no complications.

The hardest part of recovery, Lupe shared, was feeling very weak for a few weeks but not from hunger and wanting to chew.

After surgery she could only consume one ounce of fluid at a time. For 2 weeks she was to be on clear foods only, then to milky, then to pureed food and then to chunky. It would be 8 to 10 weeks before chewing could resume.

One of the scariest moments for her was being at home two weeks after surgery, finding her hand in the candy bowl, and realizing she couldn't do that.

Accompanying the surgery, there was a balanced lean protein diet to follow. Staying away from sugar, carbs, and unhealthy fats was a big part of the diet. Here are some examples of meals when it came time to chew. Breakfast consisted of a high-level protein shake. Lunch was a piece of chicken or a salad. A work time lunch may possibly be a high protein bar. Dinner might consist of a small piece of meat with a bit of green veggies or a protein shake. Lupe talked about her watch on her liquid intake to insure her water level was where it needed to be.

Lupe confessed, "I can't tell you that I did it, but a diet accompanying this surgery was given to me."

Another factor to eating after surgery was about drinking liquids. There is only so much room in a quarter of a stomach. So, it was necessary to drink 20 minutes before you eat or 20 minutes after you eat.

Q... What were the cons to your experience?
A... An important factor I later became aware of because I paid out-of-pocket. Insurance forces you to go through a certain amount of psychological evaluations. Had I known the importance of the evaluations, I would have paid for that out-of-pocket also. I would have taken the opportunity to prepare myself and understand that my weight gain was a result of an addictive personality, not what I ate. I dealt with the anatomy of it, not the psychology of it.

Q... Did you reach your goal?
A... No, I was 15 pounds shy of my goal, but I also did not follow the instructions.

Q... Why didn't you follow it?
A... I never dealt with the reason I got where I got. I am an emotional eater. I eat when I'm sad, I eat when I'm happy, I eat when I'm angry, I eat when I'm stressed....... I eat for every emotion.

Q... Let's look at the positive side to your experience. What were the pros?
A... It took me to a healthier state. At the time of my DMI as I said before, I was less than 6 months away from being a full-blown diabetic. After the surgery, within 6 months, I was healthy as a horse. It gave me back an ability to hit a reset button.

Q... Would you recommend this surgery to others?
A... Yes, and looking back, I would do it again. I don't think I would be where I am today if I had not done it.

Q... Do you have any additional thoughts for others?
A... If it is an option for someone, I'd like to suggest making sure you take the opportunity to deal with an understanding of the why you have your eating pattern. I regret that I didn't take it more seriously in the first year. All was explained to me, but I ignored it. That first year is an adaptive year of your body. You need to reach your goal at all costs, through increased exercise, change in eating behavior and truly take that year of transformation seriously. Because I did not take heed of the information available and given to me, I easily got re-acclimated into what I do day in and day out. And found ways to say, "It's okay, I'm in a good spot." And make excuses for not doing and following what was laid out for me.

Well, that ended my interview with Lupe about her surgery....but there's more....Lupe gained 40 pounds back.

Q... Lupe, what happened? What were you eating?
A... Too much... I'm a sugar person. I will drink and eat sugar. I like fried foods and sugary stuff. I like carbohydrates. I had found a way to incrementally increase my portions but not like the size they used to be before surgery. One year after surgery I went down to 164 pounds. Within the next two and a half years I went up to 198 pounds. I went back to my doctor who treats my thyroid and she was like, "What in the world did you do????" After reading me the riot act, she

considered putting me on an injectable plan. It's similar to insulin. You're supposed to gradually increase the dose until you make yourself nauseated. That's how it helps you control your over-consumption. That medication was over $1800.00 for a 30-day supply. Needless to say, that was not going to be an option, nor did I want to be nauseated all day long. So we talked about my lifestyle and my crazy work schedule and the fact that I was married with a family and a special needs child. With this, she said, "Can you pre-package some of your food? Can you try to plan your week?"

Lupe told me her immediate thought with that suggestion (which she shared with her doctor), "If I knew how to do this properly, I would have done it." She added, "I was introduced to the Optavia opportunity from a friend at church. I asked my doctor's opinion about the program and her response was that it was one of the better rated pre-packaged food plans as far as quality. She did not support it, nor prescribe it. But she was not opposed to it."

This program is pre-packaged food for the most part. It's about calorie control but it is done for you within the plan. Among other factors, the Optavia plan, with its pre-packaged meals, offers fueling bars throughout the day along with a suggested meal for dinner. With their food plan, a significant amount of water intake is essential. Lupe personally enjoyed the fueling bars. They provided a "grab and go" for her. The entire program was very convenient for her lifestyle. She lost 20 pounds in a little over a month and a half.

Lupe said, "Again, Michele, the cycle is the same. When I follow the rules it works, when I break the rules it doesn't. My experience and weight gain has always been an upfront issue. I know why I gain weight. It is no surprise. It's the amount of food I'm eating and the time in which I eat it."

With modification, Lupe feels like this diet plan can be an ongoing way of keeping her weight in check. It has helped her to be much more conscious of her portion control and intake of calories. The first 3 days, she mentioned that she was a little tired and it was a little weird getting used to the program. But when the tired feeling passed, she felt good and did not feel hungry.

She has currently modified the program to two bars, a few snacks and one meal per day, or three bars and two meals throughout the day. Lupe was pleased that presently, being off of most of the prepackaged program, she still could have portion-controlled regular food including a glass of wine.

For the last 2 months, she has maintained her weight, however she is ready to go back to the initial diet plan of the program full force, consuming the recommended amount of water, 5 fueling bars throughout the day and one meal in order to rid herself of the rest of her unwanted weight.

Q... Did you feel deprived of any foods that you enjoy on this program?
A... Not really, because I believe in living my life. I did try not to cheat; however, if I was dining out for business or a special event, I would eat what was before me.

Optavia is a multi-level marketing program, but Lupe has not looked into the business aspect of it. But what she did share was that Optavia has a great support system. You have a one-on-one coach. You can call a nutritionist on a 1-800 number through Optavia and receive personal advice. They suggest that you check with your physician concerning the given advice. There are educational videos available, and it has a worldwide community to connect with through different social networks like Facebook, Pinterest and others.

She would absolutely recommend Optavia to others. But she also recommends doing it correctly.

As you have read, Lupe has recommended both her surgery and her present experience with Optavia. As she stated in the first part of her interview, she would not be where she is today had it not been for the surgery. Surgery was the path she needed to take at that time in her life.

Lupe's final thoughts were, "I have come across people who I personally know who were looking into surgery that have been able to drop the weight using the Optavia plan. It enabled them to get to a better place without surgery."

THIS INTERVIEW WITH OLGA IS INFORMATIVE

She had her procedure done in 2014, just four years ago. When she looked into medical alternatives for her weight loss, there were three procedures that were discussed.

One was the gastric bypass, which she found to be too extreme. It created more restrictions of what your body could and could not produce. After the surgery, one would always need (not as an option, but a need) to take vitamins or supplements.

Another was a gastric ring or donut. This did not allow you to lose much weight and it was easy to gain it back.

And the third which she elected was the gastric sleeve. Your body stays the same with its basic functions. This procedure removes 75% of your stomach, simply making it smaller.

She was hospitalized for just one night and her recovery time was a week, with no complications.

I asked her about immediate results. She said she had no desire to eat. Actually, she had to force herself to eat. Her doctor reduced her calorie intake and upped her liquids two weeks prior to the procedure. Olga found this quite positive. This would help the change in her food intake not to be so drastic.

After the surgery, she likened her retraining to eating like that of a baby. She started on bland liquids and from there she went to puree and then to solids which was in about a 4-week period.

Her cravings were gone, but she wasn't sure how or why that happened. She hasn't had a desire for soda for the last 4 years. Hunger wasn't an issue, but she said the mind still wanted to chew.

Her breakfast consists of an egg and maybe a cup of coffee. Lunch was generally 5 ounces of a meat and possibly some carrots. Again, her dinner was veggies and a protein entrée. Olga said she was always full and satisfied.

She added that it was a forced learning experience. Her stomach would reject old eating habits. If she chose to eat something that her stomach was not ready to accept yet, she would feel very nauseated.

She said, "Adding a small bite of rice and beans to my plate, being Cuban, I would have to give up something else. Because remember, only 25% of my stomach is left. Drinking liquids while eating, because of the space it takes in your stomach, is a no-no. Drinking liquid should be done before or after meals. My husband said, 'I'm a cheap date these days.' When we go out to dinner, we order one meal and share."

Q... Olga, did you feel deprived?
A... No, because before surgery, I would have a large steak, a lot of rice and beans, plantains, etc. I would be so, so, full. I have the same feeling now just with smaller amounts. I have learned to make healthier choices.

I asked her what she meant by healthier choices. Oh-my-goodness, she jumped right in on this one. I had to giggle.... She said, "Healthy choices? That's easy. Stay away from fast foods. You can choose, if you must, to have a salad or have a burger, to have a burger without the bun or even choose to have half of a burger. It's a choice not to add fries or an ice cream. Maybe you'll choose to have a few fries instead of eating them all."

She finished this question with, "As a child we learned to clean our plates, but it's a healthy choice to leave some food behind."

She lost 85 pounds of her 100-pound goal. I inquired about improved health issues, and her response was, "My allergies, sinuses, blood pressure, cholesterol and diabetic issues are gone or greatly improved. My diabetes is gone, my once high blood pressure is normal, and my cholesterol levels are perfect."

Q... And, the cons to this are?
A... Hmm. There are so many positives, I have to think on this one. I wish it would have been stressed more in my psychiatric evaluation prior to surgery how important the first year was to learn how to eat properly with healthy choices. Your stomach maintains the ability to stretch. As a result, I have gained some back and I'm dealing with the struggle to lose again but the struggle is much, much, easier.

Olga finished her interview with this:
Q... Would you recommend this procedure to others?
A... Absolutely. 100%. I did gain some of my lost pounds back as I stated before. I gained not only by personal choices but also (although greatly improved) gained because of some health issues and medications. This procedure was such a great tool. (Olga stressed that it is a 'tool'.) One that you must follow. It's the best decision I ever made. It was a tool that changed my life. I know how to pull back today on wrong choices for me.

A MUST READ
A BLOG FROM TINA PETERSEN

My name is Tina Petersen. I am a mother, a retired psychotherapist, a personal trainer and group fitness instructor who loves to motivate others to be better and to do better. My passion and purpose in life is to allow the Lord to use me to draw out the goodness in others.

I am a licensed psychotherapist, with my Master's Degree in Clinical Counseling Psychology. I have worked with all different walks of life during my therapy work including children, adults, couples and families. I no longer practice at the community mental health agency I worked for; however, I do still practice one night a month at a local cancer foundation, facilitating cancer groups.

Through my work at the cancer foundation, I truly learned the value of whole food nutrition and how food can heal the human body. After leaving group one night I began praying for a solution to protect my family, specifically my husband Dan, son Gavin, and daughter Addyson from disease and illness. I knew flooding their bodies with fruits and vegetables and removing processed foods would be the answer, however, and I did not know the "how" to do this. My two-year old would not eat veggies at that time, so how could I flood his body with the good stuff? I prayed and prayed, and then the answer came!

My brother-in-law came home one weekend from New York City, gifting my husband a box of Juice Plus for his birthday: raw, vine ripened fruits, vegetables, berries, and grains that are juiced, dehydrated and put into a capsule or chewable! Juice Plus is not a traditional vitamin, it is food, carrying a nutrition label on the back of the bottle. The product is NSF certified and has research proving the many health benefits from eating it! The Lord was listening and sent this amazing solution. Amen!

For the past four years, my family has been eating Juice Plus and following a healthy lifestyle. We are healthier and happier than ever! Our immune systems are stronger, our eating habits have improved, we sleep better, our digestion is better, and our overall health continues to improve!

There are many diets and "quick fixes" out there. I personally do not believe in any of these ways. I believe making a healthy lifestyle is the only solution. What does lifestyle mean to me? It means eating clean whole foods, limiting processed foods and any activities that do not improve my health in any way. For me, lifestyle specifically includes eating mostly plant based. I no longer eat any meats; however, I do consume fish. My family does eat meat still; however, all meats are organic, grass-fed, non-GMO, hormone free meats. The foods we tend to eat come from a plant, not a bag.

Along with eating clean, I believe moving the body is essential. I fit exercise into my day, every single day. For each person, exercise means something different. The importance is that the body is in motion. Our joints, muscles, heart and brain truly benefit from exercise. We release happy hormones called endorphins when we exercise, something all humans need! Through exercise, we build more muscle, and improve our cardiovascular health, as well as our mental health. I believe in feeling strong, not skinny. Weight loss will most likely take place when committing to clean eating and exercising; however, I believe it should not be the main focus. Feeling strong and improving your fitness is the indicator of progress that I use to determine goals being met, NOT THE SCALE!

As I stated earlier, there is no magic pill or short cut out there. Once a person can commit to the basics, eating clean and exercising ... the magic starts to happen! The body and mind begin to transform, and self-love and acceptance begin to be the end result. For our family, Juice Plus has been the catalyst to our positive health changes. It has completely changed the picture of our health!

The Lord truly has a plan for each of us. I am incredibly grateful the Lord brought nutrition and fitness into my life and am even more grateful that He is using me to inspire others to take control of their health!

FAT IS YOUR FRIEND
A BLOG FROM PASTOR ANTHONY STORINO

Let me tell you my journey! In March 2017, I visited my cardiologist. I already have 4 stents. The doctor looked at my blood work and my weight and said, with a straight face, "If you don't lose weight you're going to die."

My blood work was off the charts; 300+ cholesterol, HDL of 18, LDL 250+, triglycerides 250. I said, "Doctor, I go by the guidelines you set up: no saturated fat, low cholesterol foods." Most of you know the drill. He told me, "Do yourself a favor and lay off the bread, the sugar and refined flour. Eat whole wheat and the like."

Someone gave me a book by Dr. Joseph Mercola called *Fat for Fuel*. To be honest with you, I read it. It was very technical. If I were in the health care profession, I would have understood it better. But I did follow his recommendations and started watching some of the videos on the subject.

So, let's fast forward to my May 21, 2107 *I ate my last CARB loaded meal*, at one my favorite Italian restaurants! And… I have several favorites.

So, on May 22, 2017, I started eating a ketogenic, LCHF (Low Carb High Fat) diet. It has been a journey. Almost overwhelming in the beginning. But truly, today I would not trade it for anything.

I eat 30 carbs or less in a day (Occasionally I will treat myself to more on a special occasion or something), but I am very strict in my carb counting. I eat about 125 to 140 grams of fat a day and about 80 to 110 grams of protein a day. I eat beef, chicken and eggs, fish, nuts, avocados, and leafy green veggies (spinach, brussels sprouts, kale, bok choy, asparagus, broccoli, broccoli rabe, and as a substitute mashed potato, I use mashed cauliflower).

My wife and I have learned to bake with almond flower, and with it we make bread and pizza dough. We've substituted pasta with eggplant, spaghetti squash or zucchini.

So, on my journey I have gathered a lot of followers and we do it together and share different recipes and are there to support one another. Once a month I do a seminar called "Fat Is Your Friend". We are getting ready to start a once-a-week group.

But here I am today, 54lbs. lighter. I went from 236 pounds to 182 pounds, no aches and pains, my sugar is a normal A1C from 7.1 to 5.0. My triglycerides are normal from 195 to 80. I no longer take medications. My cholesterol went down, and I am off cholesterol medication, it has gone up, but in extensive research, reading and study I have discovered that cholesterol is not the problem (you need cholesterol to survive, you brain is made up of it), but carbs from sugar are the problem. As a matter of fact, sugar is the leading cause of Alzheimer disease in the world.

Well at 236 pounds on May 22, 2017, I started LCHF and immediately started to see results. Sixty days into the LCHF my blood work came back, and all my blood numbers were in the normal range. My A1C is 5.0 and I had lost considerable weight. I feel the best I've ever felt. No more aches or pains. Contrary to what all the naysayers said, I kept with it.

I am going to be 70 years old in a few months, I walk on average 5 to 7 miles 3 times a week. I am including 2 pictures of myself, one in March 2017 at 236 pounds and one in late August at 189 pounds. Today, one year later, I am 180 pounds. I have set a goal to lose another 10 pounds. I feel great, have more energy than I ever had and no more back problems.

I am a pastor of a charismatic church on the Jersey Shore. Because I have such a great staff, I can work a 4-day week managing a beach resort, where I am on my feet from 7:00 AM until the beach closes. Prior to this I would work up at that beach and have to sit most of the day because I was out breath and my chest would hurt. After service on Sundays, I would have to go home to lay down and nap. Today, I minister 3 times a week and I work up at the beach and outdo all the younger people who are under my management; they look at me in amazement; what a great feeling.

I went from a 44-inch waist to a 34-inch waist, went from XXL to Large, and from a size 50 sports coat to a size 44.

Just one more thing. I am no longer on any medication, except for blood pressure which went from 2 pills to 1 half the milligrams.

I am so blessed to have learned about LCHF -- I am on a mission to tell everyone who is having health problems you must do this and live well and healthy. My doctor is not quite a believer yet, but he knows he cannot argue with the success I have had.

So yes, I am a LCHF Keto person and sometimes I go carnivore, meaning for 7 to 14 days only meat.

After   Before

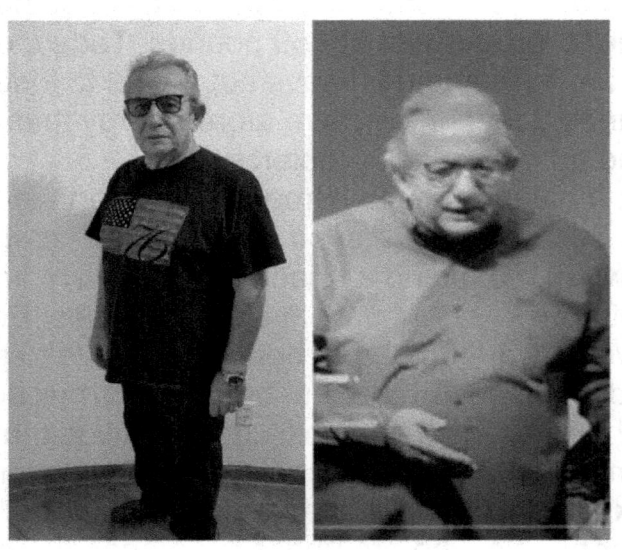

Chapter 13 -- *Can I help you?*

    E-mail me at Firstmate0825@outlook.com if you have any questions, or if you would just like to bounce some ideas my way or thoughts that you may have when starting your search.

    If you would like ideas with modifying your favorite meals or dishes, it would be my pleasure to help if I can. My goal would be to duplicate a like taste and texture, carb, calorie, sodium and cholesterol friendly dish.

    First, send a recipe. Next, let me know which of the following items you would like to see modified.

    After reviewing your request, I will be able to determine how I can assist you and promptly reply.

Carbohydrates.

Calories.

Cholesterol.

Sodium.

Sugar.

Protein.

Fiber.

Saturated fats.

Other_____

Any additional information that you would like to add.

_____

_____

Simple consultations are free via email but If you would like to proceed further on your favorite recipe, there will be a non-refundable, modest fee for the cost of the food and preparation time that will be estimated in advance. This includes the purchase of food items for the original recipe, which I will prepare and taste; plus, the purchase of the food items to make the modified recipe, which I will also prepare for quality modification.

Please note that any vulgarity or inappropriate requests will not be tolerated. You will be reported and blocked.

Chapter 14 -- *Closing Thoughts*

LET'S SUM THIS UP

Which is the healthiest, the quickest, the most practical, the cleanest and the greenest? Only you can decide which type of plan you will have success with, which one will reinforce a determination for the discipline required and the ability to follow through.

Because of ongoing research, there is always going to be a healthier, more practical and a more complete "clean and green" way, and of course, new fad diets for promised quick results.

Everyone has different strengths and weaknesses and I hope that through reading *Time to Stop the Battle (Eating with Freedom)*, you took away who you are and what's going to work for you.

Hopefully, you recognized the commonalities we all share. I'm sure there is someone, somewhere, that honestly does not enjoy those forbidden carbs of some sort, like breads and sweets. I just haven't met them yet. This common forbidden carb thread seems to be the "Biggy" in most food battles. And of course everyone has choices and life changes to deal with.

Many of the interviewees claimed more energy as a result of their plan. But note.... these claims came from completely different diets. And of course everyone had their own choices and changes to endure. This seems to be a common thread with all of them. It may not be within these pages, but if you're ready, there is a plan for you'.

So... Where do **you** start?

You have already started. You have taken the time to read this book. You know the types of food that you like and the ones you tend to overindulge in. And because you are searching, my guess is that you probably have come across a plan that seems feasible. Consider that feasible plan as you read on.

I would suggest you start with the meals and snacks that you are currently enjoying. Make a list of common meals you choose through the week for breakfast, lunch and dinner. Really look at them. Know what you're dealing with. Don't forget....snacks too.

Try not to eliminate, but instead modify. Modify them by bringing down the numbers through the many substitution I have shared throughout this book. Denying doesn't work.

You are going to change your intake of carbohydrates, fats, sodium and processed foods to some degree. Some things may increase, and some will decrease. This again is a personal choice. It truly depends on which plan you choose. For example, we substituted fat-free for whole cheeses, vegan and chicken links for pork sausage, etc. But if you feel a keto plan is the way you should go, you would want to include whole milk cheeses and pork sausage.

What is important, is to modify your overall meals. Changes need to be made, but not necessarily your food choices. Just the modifications that I have covered throughout this book.

Remember, with any plan, there are foods that have to be eaten in moderation. But not all foods. Most plans have a "free food" list or choices that allow you to comfortably have seconds.

And when you find a plan you want to try, use Goggle to help you modify your favorite meals. You can even modify any suggested meals in a chosen diet. Just make sure the numbers are the same. Be true to your taste buds.

If you are determined to follow through with your chosen plan but have one of those 'see it and eat it' kind of days, well, welcome to the humanity of dieting. It is an "ism" that happens to the most faithful of dieters. Every morning is a new start. You do get a 'do-over'.

And if you choose a plan that's not working for you, don't get discouraged. You've just learned what doesn't work for you. It's just a stepping stone away from the wrong direction that will enable you to go forward --- toward a new start!

Keep pressing forward…

God Bless you,
Hugs
Michele

---

ism = I – Self -- Me

Recipes at Your Fingertips

A quick guide by meal type for all of the recipes that I prepare. I have taken each recipe from this book and placed them here by meal and the corresponding page number to simply locate the recipe that you want to prepare.

Breakfast

Toast Fingers with Syrup	58
Oatmeal	58
Mom's Smashed Banana and Peanut Butter	58
Pancakes with Sausage Links	59
Pancake Sandwich	60
Omelets	61
Breakfast Burritos	62
Sausage, Egg 'n Cheese	63

Lunches

Ham 'n Cheddar Cheese Sandwich	66
Turkey 'n Swiss Cheese Sandwich	66
Toasty Ham 'n Cheese Melt	67
Wrap It	68
Diggity Dogs	69
Baked Beans	70
Cheeseburger Wrap	71
Simple Chicken or Tuna Salad Lettuce Wrap	72
Egg Salad	73
Chicken Fajita Wraps	74
I'm a PB2 Lover Wrap	76
Burgers	77
Cheeseburger Salad	78
Grilled Sausage Sandwich	79

Dinners

Chicken Stock	53
Spagetts with Bolognese Sause	82
Squashy Alternative for Spagetts	83
Zucchini Noodles	84
Hearty Escarole Soup	85
Chicken with Broccoli Casserole	88
Spinachy Sausage 'n Pasta	89
Sausage, Pepper 'n Onion Sub	90
Leftover Cheesy Meatball Sub	91
Another Low-Cal Sub	92
Pepper Steak Sub	93

Chicken or Turkey SOS	94
Cheesy Chicken Fritters	95
Crispy Breading	96
Spanglish Pork Chops	97
Hillbilly Chili	98
Tortilla Soup	99
Meatloaf	100
Shepherd's Pie	101
Stuffed Cabbage	102
Zitiagna	103
20 Minute Pizza	104
Meatballs	105
Stroganoff	106
Braised Country Style Pork Ribs	107
Pork Butt Steaks	108
Easy-Peasy Clam Sauce and Linguine	109
Polenta Pizza	110
Chicken Fingers	111
Sweet 'N Sour Sauce	112
Hot Fingers (or Hot Wings)	113
Pork 'N Kraut	114
Zucchini Boats	115
Taco Salad	116

Sides, Sauces 'N Snacks

G-Moms' Pepper Sauce	117
Buttery Sweet Potatoes	118
Butternut Nuggets	119
Cauli Mash	120
Underground Medley	121
Broccoli Rabe	122
Roasted Roma Tomatoes	123
Steamed Veggies	124
Snacks	125
Pepperoni Chips	126

Dessert Time

Ricotta Cups	127
Wintery Warm Peaches	129
Fresh Strawberry Delight	130
1-2-3 Apple Pie	131
30-Second Mug Cake	132
Michelly's' Cheesecake	133
Crusty Crumbs	134
Key Lime Pie	135

Brown Sugar	136
Oatmeal Raisin Cookies	137
Carrot Cake	138
Cream Cheese Icing	139

www.ingramcontent.com/pod-product-compliance
Lightning Source LLC
Chambersburg PA
CBHW070536090426
42735CB00013B/3002